HANDBOOK
of PEDIATRIC
ANESTHESIA

NOTICE

a Lange medical book

HANDBOOK of PEDIATRIC ANESTHESIA

Editors

Philipp J. Houck, MD
Assistant Professor of Anesthesiology
Division of Pediatric Anesthesia
Department of Anesthesiology
Director of Pediatric Liver Transplant Anesthesia
New York Presbyterian-Morgan Stanley Children's Hospital
Columbia University Medical Center
New York, New York

Manon Haché, MD
Assistant Professor of Anesthesiology
Division of Pediatric Anesthesia
Department of Anesthesiology
Director of Pediatric Trauma Anesthesia
New York Presbyterian-Morgan Stanley Children's Hospital
Columbia University Medical Center
New York, New York

Lena S. Sun, MD
Emanuel M. Papper Professor of Pediatric Anesthesiology
Chief, Division of Pediatric Anesthesia
Vice Chair, Department of Anesthesiology
New York Presbyterian-Morgan Stanley Children's Hospital
Columbia University Medical Center
New York, New York

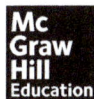

Mc
Graw
Hill
Education

New York   Chicago   San Francisco   Athens   London   Madrid   Mexico City
Milan   New Delhi   Singapore   Sydney   Toronto

Handbook of Pediatric Anesthesia

1 2 3 4 5 6 7 8 9 0 DOC/DOC 18 17 16 15 14

ISBN 978-0-07-176935-8
MHID 0-07-176935-8

This book was set in Minion Pro by MPS Limited.
The editors were Brian Belval and Robert Pancotti.
The production supervisor was Catherine H. Saggese.
Project management was provided by Vipra Fauzdar, MPS Limited.
The cover designer was Thomas De Pierro.
Front cover image: photographed by Anton Gottlob-Schoenenberger.
RR Donnelley was the printer and binder.

This book is printed on acid-free paper.

Library of Congress Cataloging-in-Publication Data

Handbook of pediatric anesthesia / editors, Philipp J. Houck, Manon Haché, Lena S. Sun.
    p. ; cm.
  ISBN 978-0-07-176935-8 (pbk: alk. paper)—ISBN 0-07-176935-8 (pbk : alk. paper)
  I. Houck, Philipp J., editor. II. Haché, Manon, editor. III. Sun, Lena S., editor.
  [DNLM: 1. Anesthesia—methods. 2. Pediatrics—methods. WO 440]
  RD139
  617.9'6798—dc23
                                                          2014020123

McGraw-Hill Education books are available at special quantity discounts to use as premiums and sales promotions or for use in corporate training programs. To contact a representative, please visit the Contact Us pages at www.mhprofessional.com.

The editors and authors of this Handbook would like to acknowledge all of our colleagues, patients, and our families for their support and encouragement who made this Handbook a reality.

CONTENTS

Part 5: Neuro

Part 6: Hematology/Oncology

Part 7: Gastrointestinal Diseases

Part 8: Metabolic Diseases

x   Contents

Appendix

Gracie M. Almeida-Chen, MD, MPH
Assistant Professor of Anesthesiology
Division of Pediatric Anesthesia
Department of Anesthesiology
New York Presbyterian-Morgan Stanley
    Children's Hospital
Columbia University Medical Center
New York, New York

Anthony J. Clapcich, MD
Associate Professor of Anesthesiology
Division of Pediatric Anesthesia
Department of Anesthesiology
Director of Difficult Airway Simulation
    Program
Director of Pediatric Cardiothoracic
    Anesthesia
New York Presbyterian-Morgan Stanley
    Children's Hospital
Columbia University Medical Center
New York, New York

Radhika Dinavahi, MD
Anesthesiologist
Miller Children's Hospital/Long Beach
    Memorial Hospital
Long Beach, California

Manon Haché, MD
Assistant Professor of Anesthesiology
Division of Pediatric Anesthesia
Department of Anesthesiology
Director of Pediatric Trauma Anesthesia
New York Presbyterian-Morgan Stanley
    Children's Hospital
Columbia University Medical Center
New York, New York

Philipp J. Houck, MD
Assistant Professor of Anesthesiology
Division of Pediatric Anesthesia
Department of Anesthesiology
Director of Pediatric Liver Transplant
    Anesthesia
New York Presbyterian-Morgan Stanley
    Children's Hospital
Columbia University Medical Center
New York, New York

Caleb Ing, MD, MS
Assistant Professor of Anesthesiology
Division of Pediatric Anesthesia
Department of Anesthesiology
New York Presbyterian-Morgan Stanley
    Children's Hospital
Columbia University Medical Center
New York, New York

E. Heidi Jerome, MD
Associate Professor of Anesthesiology
    and Pediatrics
Division of Pediatric Anesthesia
Department of Anesthesiology
Medical Director of Therapeutic and
    Interventional Imaging Unit
New York Presbyterian-Morgan Stanley
    Children's Hospital
Columbia University Medical Center
New York, New York

Robert Kazim, MD
Professor of Anesthesiology
Division of Pediatric Anesthesia
Clinical Director, Division of Pediatric
    Anesthesia
Vice Chair for Pediatric Clinical Affairs
Department of Anesthesiology
New York Presbyterian-Morgan Stanley
    Children's Hospital
Columbia University Medical Center
New York, New York

Riva R. Ko, MD
Assistant Professor of Anesthesiology
Division of Pediatric Anesthesia
Department of Anesthesiology
Co-Director of Pediatric Orthopedic
    Anesthesia
New York Presbyterian-Morgan Stanley
    Children's Hospital
Columbia University Medical Center
New York, New York

Tatiana Kubacki, MD
Assistant Professor of Anesthesiology
Division of Pediatric Anesthesia
Department of Anesthesiology
New York Presbyterian-Morgan Stanley
    Children's Hospital
Columbia University Medical Center
New York, New York

Susan Y. Lei, MD
Assistant Professor of Anesthesiology
Division of Pediatric Anesthesia
Department of Anesthesiology
New York Presbyterian-Morgan Stanley
    Children's Hospital
Columbia University Medical Center
New York, New York

Susumu Ohkawa, MD
Staff Anesthesiologist
Lenox Hill Hospital
New York, New York

Leila M. Pang, MD
Ngai-Jubilee Professor of
   Anesthesiology
Vice Chair for Resident Education
Department of Anesthesiology
New York Presbyterian-Morgan Stanley
   Children's Hospital
Columbia University Medical Center
New York, New York

Teeda Pinyavat, MD
Assistant Professor of Anesthesiology
Division of Pediatric Anesthesia
Department of Anesthesiology
Co-Director of Pediatric Orthopedic
   Anesthesia
New York Presbyterian-Morgan Stanley
   Children's Hospital
Columbia University Medical Center
New York, New York

Neeta R. Saraiya, MD
Assistant Professor of Anesthesiology
Division of Pediatric Anesthesia
Department of Anesthesiology
Director of Student Anesthesia
   Internship Program
New York Presbyterian-Morgan Stanley
   Children's Hospital
Columbia University Medical Center
New York, New York

John M. Saroyan, MD
Medical Director
BAYADA Hospice
Norwich, Vermont

William S. Schechter, MD
Professor of Anesthesiology and
   Pediatrics
Division of Pediatric Anesthesia
Department of Anesthesiology
Director of Pediatric Pain Medicine and
   Advanced Care Medicine
New York Presbyterian-Morgan Stanley
   Children's Hospital
Columbia University Medical Center
New York, New York

Arthur J. Smerling, MD
Associate Professor of Pediatrics and
   Anesthesiology
Medical Director of Pediatric Cardiac
   Critical Care Unit
New York Presbyterian-Morgan Stanley
   Children's Hospital
Columbia University Medical Center
New York, New York

Lena S. Sun, MD
Emanuel M. Papper Professor of
   Pediatric Anesthesiology
Chief, Division of Pediatric Anesthesia
Vice Chair, Department of
   Anesthesiology
New York Presbyterian-Morgan Stanley
   Children's Hospital
Columbia University Medical Center
New York, New York

Mary E. Tresgalio, DNP, MPH, FNP-BC
Assistant Professor of Nursing
School of Nursing
Columbia University Medical Center
New York, New York

PREFACE

The pediatric anesthesiology faculty at Columbia University Medical Center has put together this book as a guide to the practice of clinical anesthesia in neonates, infants, children, and adolescents. The authors are clinicians with considerable experience in the practice of pediatric anesthesiology. They are also teachers of pediatric anesthesiology. Their daily work includes the education and training of residents and fellows in pediatric anesthesiology in a major academic teaching hospital. This book is not "Pediatric Anesthesia for Dummies." Rather, the authors have organized it as a collection of common and important conditions in children. For each condition, the authors outline the pathophysiology, key perioperative considerations, and important management issues. We hope that residents and practicing physicians will find the book useful as they plan to provide anesthesia care for children.

1 INTRODUCTION

Robert Kazim, MD

This introduction will highlight the key physiological, anatomical, and pharmacological concepts that novices in pediatric anesthesiology will find helpful for understanding current practice in this field.

THE INFANT AIRWAY

Seven anatomical features distinguish the infant airway from the adult.

1. The tongue is large in relation to the oral cavity, predisposing infants to airway obstruction and challenging intubation. Infants are obligate nasal breathers until 3-5 months of life. Obstruction of the anterior and/or posterior nares (secondary to nasal congestion, stenosis, or choanal atresia) may cause asphyxia.
2. The larynx is positioned higher in the neck (C3-C4) than in adults (C5-C6), allowing for simultaneous nasal breathing and swallowing.
    The larynx creates an acute angulation at the base of the tongue, creating the impression of an anterior larynx. Use of a straight laryngoscope blade to lift the base of the tongue and epiglottis, along with external laryngeal pressure, can aid in viewing the larynx during intubation.
3. The epiglottis is Ω-shaped and protrudes posteriorly over the larynx at a 45° angle; it may be difficult to lift during laryngoscopy.
4. The vocal cords attach anteriorly, which is more caudal and predisposes to catching the tip of the endotracheal tube in the anterior commissure during intubation.
5. The cricoid cartilage is conically shaped and is the narrowest portion of the upper airway (true for the first decade of life) (Fig. 1-1).
    Precise endotracheal tube sizing is critical to avoid cricoid edema and postintubation croup. A pressure leak should be no greater than 18-20 cm H_2O. Newer high-volume–low-pressure cuffed endotracheal tubes for infants avoid repeated laryngoscopies to determine the most appropriate endotracheal tube size.
    Given that resistance to airflow is inversely proportional to radius to the fourth power, a 1-mm reduction in airway diameter increases resistance to airflow by 16-fold in the infant airway.
6. The tonsils and adenoids are small in the neonate but reach maximal size in the first 4-5 years of age. Use of continuous positive pressure and/or an oral airway will commonly overcome this obstruction.

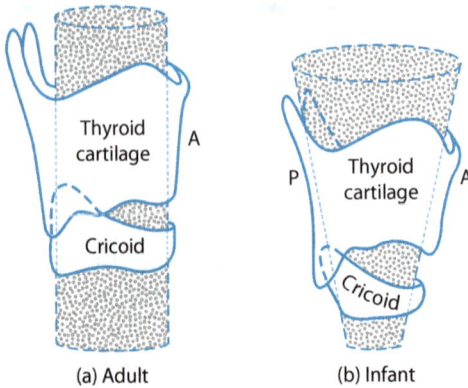

FIGURE 1-1 Schematic of an adult (a) and infant (b) airway. A, Anterior; P, Posterior. [Reprinted from Cote CJ, Todres ID. The pediatric airway. In: Ryan JF, Todres ID, Cote CJ, et al, eds. *A Practice of Anesthesia for Infants and Children*. Philadelphia, PA: WB Saunders; 1986:35-58, with permission from Elsevier.]

7. The occiput is large. When the infant is placed on a flat surface, extreme neck flexion will cause airway obstruction. A small roll placed behind the baby's shoulders will reduce neck flexion and aid in maintaining the airway.

PEDIATRIC RESPIRATORY PHYSIOLOGY

LOWER AIRWAY

The alveolar bed is incompletely developed at birth; mature alveoli are seen at 5 weeks of age, with alveolar multiplication with adult morphology being reached by 8 years of life (Table 1-1). Infant lung compliance is

TABLE 1-1	RESPIRATORY SYSTEM DEVELOPMENT
Age	
24 weeks gestation	Gas exchanging surface forms Surfactant production begins
Newborn	Decreased reserve because of: • Increased oxygen consumption • Decreased FRC
60 weeks postconception	Increased risk of postoperative apnea in premature infants until this age
8 years	Number of alveoli reach adult values
10 years	Fully muscular pulmonary arteries are seen at the alveolar duct level
19 years	Fully muscular pulmonary arteries are seen at the level of the alveoli

extremely high due to the absence of elastic fibers; it resembles the emphysematous lung. It is prone to airway collapse and premature airway closure secondary to low elastic recoil.

The cartilaginous rib cage and poorly developed intercostal muscles result in a highly compliant chest wall, leading to inefficient ventilation. The circular configuration of the rib cage (which is ellipsoid in adults) and the horizontally attached diaphragm (which is oblique in adults) lead to poor respiratory mechanics. The chest wall begins to stiffen at 6 months of age, improving the outward recoil of the chest wall.

The diaphragm has fewer Type I muscle fibers (sustained twitch, highly oxidative, and fatigue resistant) and is susceptible to fatigue. The adult diaphragm contains 55%, the neonate 25%, and the preterm only 10% Type I fibers.

LUNG VOLUMES

Functional residual capacity (FRC) in the spontaneously breathing infant is dynamically maintained at 40% of total lung capacity (similar to adults). See Table 1-2. The following mechanisms play a role in dynamically maintaining FRC in the *awake* infant:

- Termination of the expiratory phase before the lung volume reaches FRC, "auto-PEEP"
- Glottic closure during the expiratory phase (grunting), maintaining lung volumes
- Diaphragmatic braking: diminished diaphragmatic activity extending to the expiratory phase
- Tonic activity of the diaphragmatic and intercostal muscles, stiffening the chest wall and maintaining higher lung volumes

Dynamic control of FRC is abolished in the *anesthetized* child. Under apneic conditions, the FRC has been estimated to be reduced to 10% of total lung capacity. The reduced FRC results in reduced intrapulmonary oxygen reserve and rapid hypoxemia in the infant.

TABLE 1-2   AGE-DEPENDENT RESPIRATORY VALUES

	Neonate	Infant	Child/Adult
Tidal volume (mL/kg)	6-8	6-8	7-8
Respiratory frequency (bpm)	30-50	20-30	12-16
Minute ventilation (mL/kg/min)	200-260	175-185	80-100
Functional residual capacity (mL/kg)	22-25	25-30	30-45
Total lung capacity (mL/kg)	60	70	80
Metabolic rate (mL/kg/min)	6-8		3-4

NEONATAL APNEA

Apnea is defined as cessation of breathing for 10-15 seconds and can be associated with bradycardia and loss of muscle tone. Apnea is common in premature infants (defined as gestational age <38 weeks) and is related to immature respiratory control mechanisms. This phenomenon is rare in full-term infants. Both theophylline and caffeine have effectively reduced apneic episodes in these infants. Exposure to respiratory depressants, such as inhaled agents, opioids, and benzodiazepines, all induce apnea in this population.

Premature infants less than 58-60 weeks postconceptual age have been shown to be at greater risk of postanesthetic apnea. Apneic episodes have been described up to 12 hours postoperatively.

Use of a regional anesthetic technique, ie, spinal anesthesia, has been advocated in this population, although it has not been shown to reduce the incidence of apnea. Therefore, the need for observation in the perioperative period is not dependent on the anesthetic technique.

NEONATAL HYPOXEMIA

Respiratory control is poorly developed in neonates and preterm infants.

- Increased metabolic demand.
- Prone to upper airway obstruction.
- Immature respiratory control and irregular breathing.
- Hypoxia transiently increases then depresses ventilation.
- Hypoxia depresses hypercapneic ventilatory response.
- Anesthetics abolish mechanisms to maintain FRC.

NEONATAL RENAL FUNCTION

Renal components are incompletely developed at birth, although the formation of nephrons is complete at 36 weeks gestation. Rapid maturation occurs during the first month of life, then these components continue to fully mature over the first year of life:

- Reduced glomerular filtration rate (GFR)—25% of adult
- Inadequate tubular function (adult values reached after 2 years of age)

Neonates have difficulty with *both* volume loading and volume depletion. Volume depletion, though, has more serious implications. Sodium balance is directly related to intake. The administration of sodium-free solutions may lead rapidly to hyponatremia.

BODY COMPOSITION

Water constitutes 75% of the weight of a neonate as compared with 65% of that of a 12-month-old infant and 55% of that of an adult. The reduction in total body water is accompanied by a shift in the distribution of

TABLE 1-3   ASSESSMENT OF HYDRATION/EXTENT OF DEHYDRATION

Signs/Symptoms	Dehydration (%)	Fluid Deficit (mL/kg)
Thirsty, restless	5	50
Poor tissue turgor, sunken fontanelle	10	100
Orthostatic, oliguric, comatose	15	150

fluid from extracellular to intracellular. Fat represents 16% of the body weight of a neonate and increases to 23% by 12 months of age.

Increased fluid requirements occur with:

- Increased metabolic rate
- Increased insensible fluid loss
- Increased obligatory fluid loss

See Table 1-3 for a summary of hydration assessment.

INFANT FLUID REPLACEMENT

Typically 50% of the deficit is replaced over the first hour, with the remaining deficit being replaced over the next 2 hours. Maintenance fluids can be calculated using the 4/2/1 rule.

Surgical procedures involving only mild tissue trauma may entail third space losses of 3-4 mL/kg/h. This ranges up to 10 mL/kg/h in very large abdominal procedures.

VITAL SIGNS

Changes in heart rate, respiratory rate, and blood pressure as the child ages are summarized in Table 1-4.

TABLE 1-4   TYPICAL VITAL SIGNS

Age	Heart Rate	Systolic BP	Diastolic BP	Respiratory Rate
Preterm, first day	120	50	35	60
Full term, first day	120	65	45	50
1 month	160	95	55	40
3 months	140	95	60	30
1 year	125	95	60	24
3 years	100	100	65	24
8 years	80	105	70	22
12 years	75	115	75	18

NEONATAL HYPOGLYCEMIA

Hypoglycemia in the first 3 days of life is defined in the preterm infant as BS <20 mg/dL and in the full-term infant as BS <30 mg/dL. After 3 days of age, blood glucose levels should be >40 mg/dL. Neonates have limited hepatic glycogen stores, leading to deficient gluconeogenesis. When these stores are rapidly depleted during increases in metabolic demand, hypoglycemia ensues.

In addition to limited gluconeogenesis, other causes of hypoglycemia include:

- Increased insulin secretion (Beckwith/Wiedemann)
- Perinatal hypoxemia
- Sepsis
- Toxemia of pregnancy

Children at greatest risk for hypoglycemic episodes include:

- Preterm neonates
- Term infants
- Small for gestation infants
- Infants of diabetic mothers
- Infants receiving total parenteral nutrition (TPN)

Signs and symptoms of hypoglycemia include:

- Jitteriness
- Cyanosis
- Apnea
- Lethargy
- Hypotonia
- Seizures

Treatment is critical to prevent neurologic impairment. Use slow IV administration of a 250-500-mg/kg glucose bolus followed by an infusion of D10W in 0.45NS at 65-85 mL/kg for 24 hours, monitoring glucose level to avoid rebound hypoglycemia.

Monitor blood glucose levels to avoid hyperglycemia and a hyperosmolar state, intraventricular hemorrhage, osmotic diuresis and dehydration, and further release of insulin.

INFANT TEMPERATURE REGULATION

The newborn is a homeotherm—compensatory mechanisms exist, but they regulate only within a limited temperature range (Table 1-5). The newborn is easily overwhelmed by decreases in environmental temperature. This is compounded by small size, large surface area to volume ratio (especially the head, which is 20% of the surface area compared with 9%

TABLE 1-5	INFANT TEMPERATURE REGULATION	
	Neutral Temperature*	Critical Temperature†
Preterm infant	34°C	28°C
Term infant	32°C	23°C
Adult	28°C	1°C

*Neutral temperature: the ambient temperature that results in minimal oxygen consumption.
†Critical temperature: the temperature below which the unanesthetized patient cannot maintain normal core temperature.

in the adult), thin skin, and limited fat stores. Thermal conductance, which is heat loss through skin, is inevitable.

The main mechanism for temperature regulation in the newborn period is nonshivering thermogenesis, also referred to as metabolism of brown fat. Brown fat differentiates in the fetus at between 26 and 30 weeks and makes up 2-6% of infant total body weight. These cells have an abundant vascular supply and receive innervation from the beta-adrenergic system. With exposure to a cold environment, the baby responds with increased norepinephrine production; brown fat metabolism ensues, with the production of heat.

Stores of brown fat decline during the first 6 months of life with a transition to a more adult response to alterations in temperature: shivering.

One problem with the release of norepinephrine is the end organ effect. Norepinephrine produces increased oxygen metabolism and both pulmonary and peripheral vasoconstriction, with a predisposition to right-to-left shunting and hypoxemia. The peripheral vasoconstriction produces mottling. It is therefore incumbent on the anesthesiologist to maintain the infant's temperature as outlined below.

- Transport the infant in a heated "isolette."
- Elevate room temperature to 26.6°C or 80°F for neonates.
- Use heating lamps and forced air warming.
- Warm fluids and blood products.
- Maintain low fresh gas flows and heat-moisture exchanger.
- Use protective wrap for extremities and head.

INHALATIONAL ANESTHESIA IN PEDIATRIC PATIENTS

Induction using inhalational agents is more rapid in infants as compared to adults.

There are *four* explanations for this:

- Increased alveolar ventilation to FRC ratio (infant 5:1 vs adult 1.4:1).
- Increased distribution of cardiac output to highly perfused, vessel-rich organs such as the brain and the heart.

- Increased brain mass and reduced muscle mass.
- Potent agents have reduced solubility in infants. The influence of hematocrit, hemoglobin type, and plasma protein on blood-gas solubility coefficients is not clear.

INDUCTION WITH INTRACARDIAC SHUNT

Intracardiac shunts, or ventricular septal defects (VSD), alter uptake of the inhalational agents. This is especially true for the more insoluble agents like N_2O.

Right → Left shunts slow uptake and prolong induction

Note: If cardiac function is depressed, it may be equally difficult to clear an anesthetic and resuscitate the heart and the patient.

Left → Right shunts are dependent on the size of the shunt

A large shunt (>80%) increases the rate of transfer of anesthetic to blood and therefore speeds induction.
A small shunt (<50%) has a negligible effect on induction.

MINIMUM ALVEOLAR CONCENTRATION CHANGES WITH AGE

The minimum alveolar concentration (MAC) increases progressively through the first month of life, followed by a gradual decline after 6 months of life (Fig. 1-2).

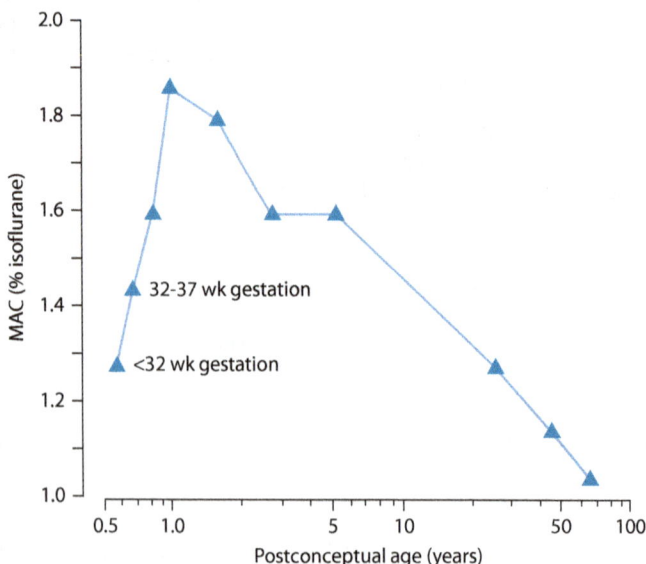

FIGURE 1-2 Age and the MAC of isoflurane from premature infants to adults. [From LeDez KM, Lerman J. The minimum alveolar concentration (MAC) of isoflurane in preterm neonates. *Anesthesiology.* 1987;67:301-307.]

SUCCINYLCHOLINE IN CHILDREN

The structure and function of the neuromuscular system is incompletely developed at birth. The margin of safety for neurotransmission is reduced in neonates.

- Conduction velocity increases with nerve fiber myelination.
- Slow-contracting muscles are progressively converted to fast contracting muscles.
- Synaptic transmission is slow.
- During repetitive stimulation, fade occurs because of a limited rate of acetylcholine release.

Succinylcholine, a depolarizing agonist, given intravenously or intramuscularly, is useful for rapid tracheal intubation and for treatment of laryngospasm. Features in infants and children include:

- Dose requirement is increased based on weight.
- Duration of action is unaffected despite reduced pseudocholinesterase activity.
- Both increased dose and limited duration appear to be due to rapid redistribution into a larger ECF volume.
- There is no phase II block on first dose.

PEDIATRIC CONTRAINDICATIONS OF SUCCINYLCHOLINE

Contraindications are similar to those in adults with one notable exception: the myopathic child. The FDA attempted to limit the use of succinylcholine because of a number of hyperkalemic cardiac arrests in children with unrecognized myopathies.

Side effects of succinylcholine are as follows:

- Cardiac arrhythmias: bradycardia, asystole, and ventricular fibrillation
- Hyperkalemia
- Postanesthetic myalgias
- Pulmonary edema
- Increased gastric, intraocular, and intracranial pressure
- Associated masseter stiffness, spasm, and malignant hyperthermia

ROCURONIUM

Rocuronium, a nondepolarizing antagonist, is considered a long-acting relaxant in infants, especially in neonates. A larger volume of distribution and slower clearance results in a prolonged neuromuscular block in infants (56 minutes vs 26 minutes in children). Onset time is slightly faster in infants. The duration of action is markedly prolonged when repeated doses are administered.

Neuromuscular function must be evaluated carefully to avoid hypoventilation-related acidosis and potentiation of relaxant. Observe the infant prior to induction (muscle tone, depth of respiration, and vigor of cry) and aim for return of this function postoperatively. Useful clinical signs include the ability to flex arms and lift legs, inspiratory force less than -25 cm H_2O, and crying vital capacity greater than 15 mL/kg. The neostigmine requirement is less in children. The onset of edrophonium is 2-3 minutes faster than that of neostigmine.

ORAL PREMEDICATION IN PEDIATRICS

Benzodiazepine derivatives are widely used for premedicating children. They are given to calm patients, allay anxiety, and diminish the recall of perianesthetic events. At low doses, minimal drowsiness and cardiovascular or respiratory depression are produced. Nausea or vomiting is rare.

Midazolam is a short-acting, water-soluble molecule with a half-life of 2 hours. It is currently the most widely used premedication because of its rapid uptake and elimination. After oral administration, there is incomplete absorption and extensive first-pass hepatic extraction, explaining the need for administration of high oral doses.

Other features include:

- Peak plasma concentrations in 53 minutes
- No increase in gastric pH or residual volume
- A calmer child
- Acceptable taste for most children
- Fewer behavioral changes than in an unpremedicated child
- Does not affect the time to recovery

Fentanyl Oralet is most effective when absorbed via the oral mucosa, not swallowed, since the first-pass metabolism through the liver is high. The effect is dose-dependent, with signs of sedation in 10 minutes after receiving 10-15 µg/kg. Desaturation and preoperative nausea are minimized if the child is brought to the OR within 10 minutes of completion of the Oralet. In doses greater than 15 µg/kg, there is an increased incidence of nausea, vomiting, pruritis, and desaturation.

REGIONAL ANESTHESIA

Advantages

- Faster awakening; reduced anesthetic requirement
- Autonomic nervous system suppression
- Limb immobilization perioperatively
- Reduced stress response

Indications

- Premature infants (<58-60 weeks prematurity)
- "Floppy" infants with neuromuscular disease
- Infants with chronic pulmonary disease
- Children at risk for malignant hyperthermia
- Older children who wish to remain awake

Contraindications

- Infection at site
- Coagulopathy
- Anatomical anomaly like spina bifida

LOCAL ANESTHETICS

Children are *not* more resistant to local anesthetic toxicity than adults:

- Decreased albumin and α-1-acid glycoprotein, both responsible for binding local anesthetics
- Reduced hepatic degradation and therefore a slower rate of elimination
- Younger infants exhibit greater free fraction of local anesthetic

  Dosing for infants <6 months and <10 kg needs to be adjusted.
  Anatomical differences of the lower central nervous system (CNS) in neonates, infants, and adults are described in Table 1-6.

COMMONLY USED TECHNIQUES

Spinal in the Neonate

- Position: sitting or lateral decubitus; support neck and administer oxygen
- Drug: Bupivacaine 0.75% 0.8 mg/kg if weight is less than 5 kg, 0.5 mg/kg if weight is over 5 kg; tetracaine (0.6-1 mg/kg with epinephrine wash) (epinephrine wash: fill and empty syringe with epinephrine 1 mg/mL); 22g spinal needle; distance from skin to subarachnoid space <1 cm in preterm infant
- Duration: 45-60 minutes

TABLE 1-6   ANATOMICAL DIFFERENCES OF LOWER CNS

	Neonate	Infant	Adult
Low end spinal cord	L3	L1	L1
Low end dural sac	S4	S2	S2
Cerebrospinal fluid (CSF) volume (mL/kg)	4	3	2
Epidural fat	Loose		Firm

Complications

- Total spinal
- Apnea
- Bradycardia

Twenty-four hour observation is mandatory in high-risk infants even after spinal anesthetic.

Caudal Block

- Locate the posterior superior iliac spines.
- Palpate the sacral cornu of the hiatus—two bony ridges approximately 0.5-1 cm apart (Fig. 1-3).
- The space between the sacrum and the coccyx may be mistaken for the sacral hiatus.
- The sacral hiatus represents failed fusion of the S5 vertebral arch.

Use a 22g angiocatheter or 22g regional anesthesia needle, insert it at 45°, then flatten the angle of advance 3-5 mm and advance the plastic catheter (Fig. 1-4). The catheter can be taped in place for longer procedures to give more local anesthetics after the conclusion of the procedure.

Drugs: 0.1-0.25% bupivacaine, maximum of 1 mL/kg; add 1-2 µg/kg of clonidine if a prolonged effect is desired.

Contraindications

- Any suspicion of a tethered cord, ie, a sacral dimple
- Same contraindications as for any other neuraxial technique

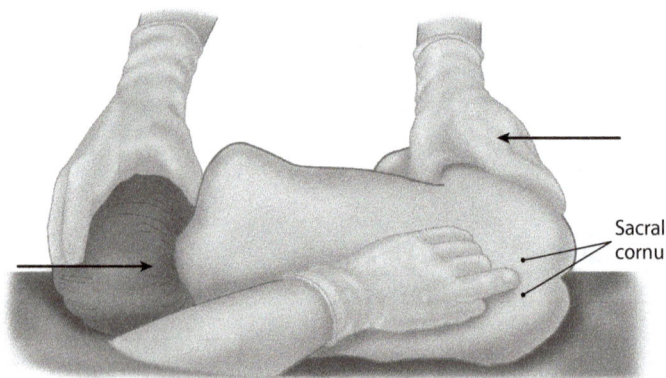

Sacral cornu

FIGURE 1-3 Positioning an anesthetized child for caudal block and palpation for the sacral hiatus. An assistant gently helps flex the spine. [From Butterworth JF, Mackey DC, Wasnick JD. *Morgan and Mikhail's Clinical Anesthesiology*. 5th ed. New York, NY: McGraw-Hill; Figure 45-20.]

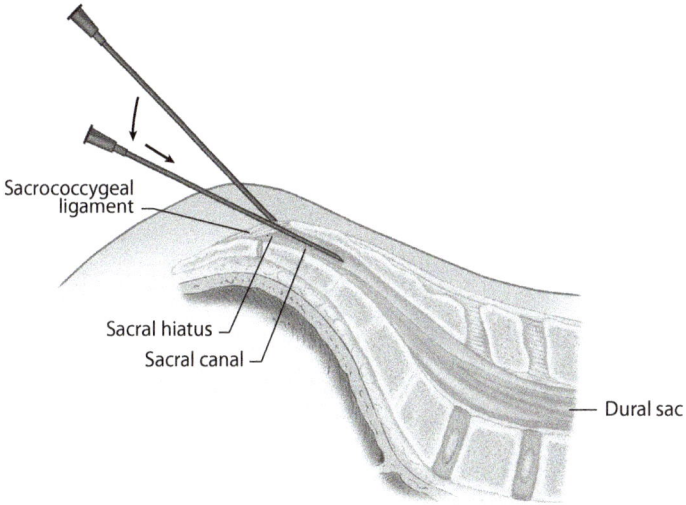

Sacrococcygeal ligament

Sacral hiatus

Sacral canal

Dural sac

FIGURE 1-4 Caudal block. [From Butterworth JF, Mackey DC, Wasnick JD. *Morgan and Mikhail's Clinical Anesthesiology.* 5th ed. New York, NY: McGraw-Hill; Figure 45-21.]

Complications

- Hematoma and infection
- Vascular puncture
- Dural puncture, especially in the very small child
- Systemic toxicity: seizures, then cardiac arrest
- Hypotension

PART 1

AIRWAY

2 TONSILLECTOMY AND ADENOIDECTOMY IN A PATIENT WITH OBSTRUCTIVE SLEEP APNEA

Gracie M. Almeida-Chen, MD, MPH

YOUR PATIENT

A 5-year-old with obstructive sleep apnea presents for tonsillectomy and adenoidectomy.

PREOPERATIVE CONSIDERATIONS

Sleep apnea is defined as a pause in breathing during sleep lasting ≥10 seconds and accompanied by at least a 4% decline in oxygen saturation from baseline despite continued respiratory efforts. Hypopnea is defined as an incomplete reduction of airflow lasting ≥10 seconds, with 50% or more reduction in tidal volume. The Apnea-Hypopnea Index is the number of apnea and hypopnea occurrences per hour during sleep (see Table 2-1). Obstructive sleep apnea (OSA) is defined as the repetition of these apneic or hypopneic spells ≥5 times per hour with symptoms associated with sleep-disordered breathing (eg, daytime hypersomnolence, cor pulmonale, and polycythemia).

The essential feature of OSA in children is increased airway resistance during sleep. Adenotonsillar hypertrophy, allergic rhinitis, turbinate hypertrophy, deviated septum, and maxillary constriction can cause airway narrowing in children. Other factors include abnormal central arousal disorder, abnormal bony anatomy, disordered neural control of airway caliber or sensation, and decreased pharyngeal tone in patients

TABLE 2-1   A SEVERITY RANKING SYSTEM BASED ON POLYSOMNOGRAPHY

	Apnea-Hypopnea Index	Oxygen Saturation Nadir
Normal	0-1	>92
Mild OSA	2-4	
Moderate OSA	5-9	
Severe OSA	>10	<80

Source: Schwengel DA, Sterni LM, Tunkel DE, Heitiller ES. Perioperative Management of Children with Obstructive Sleep Apnea. *Anesth Analg.* 2009; 109:65.

with neuromuscular conditions such as may be seen in certain types of cerebral palsy. There is an increased incidence of OSA among children with syndromes affecting their upper airway (mandibular hypoplasia in Treacher Collins or Pierre Robin syndrome; maxillary hypoplasia in Crouzon, Apert, or Pfeiffer syndrome; relative macroglossia in Down syndrome). Therefore, OSA is often a multifactorial disorder with overlapping influences that together predispose the patient to obstructed breathing.

Some 1-3% of children have OSA, and morbidities associated with OSA include symptoms of habitual problems (pauses, snorts, and gasps), daytime behavioral problems, enuresis, disturbed sleep, and daytime somnolence. It may result in a significant degree of hypercarbia and hypoxemia, leading to neurocognitive impairment, failure to thrive, dyspnea, systemic or pulmonary hypertension, and even death from cor pulmonale or arrhythmias.

The peak incidence of OSA occurs between 2 and 6 years of age and is related to when a physiological enlargement of tonsils and adenoids has occurred relative to the midfacial skeleton, which significantly expands from 6 years of age.

Key questions to ask parents during the preoperative evaluation:

- Does your child have difficulty breathing during sleep?
- Have you observed symptoms of apnea?
- Have you observed sweating while your child sleeps?
- Does your child have restless sleep?
- Does your child breathe through his/her mouth when awake?
- Are you worried about your child's breathing at night?
- Do you have any family history of obstructive sleep apnea, sudden infant death syndrome, or apparent life-threatening events?
- Does your child have behavioral problems?

Overnight polysomnography is the gold standard for the diagnosis of OSA. Overnight home pulse oximetry also provides a useful stratification of severity and may predict postoperative complications. For example, pediatric patients with significant OSA, defined as 85% or less oxygen saturation, have an increased sensitivity to opioids. Children with an oxygen saturation nadir of <85% on polysomnography required half the morphine dose needed by those with less desaturation to achieve the same level of analgesia.

Cardiac evaluation, specifically echocardiography, is recommended for any child with signs of right ventricular dysfunction, systemic hypertension, or multiple episodes of desaturation below 70%.

Noninvasive nasal positive-pressure ventilation is a common medical treatment for OSA in children. Children with very severe OSA who are at risk for persistent OSA and those with cardiovascular complications from OSA should be considered for preoperative continuous positive airway pressure/bilevel positive airway pressure (CPAP/BiPAP) therapy. Effective CPAP/BiPAP therapy may improve pulmonary hypertension and reduce the patient's surgical risks. The child's preoperative CPAP/BiPAP regimen can also be used in postoperative care.

Adenotonsillectomy is the surgical treatment of choice for children with OSA.

ANESTHETIC MANAGEMENT

- Induction of anesthesia with volatile anesthetics results in airway collapse from relaxation of the genioglossus muscle, thus placing the OSA patient at high risk for airway obstruction. Positioning in an upright or lateral position, use of a jaw thrust maneuver, delivery of positive pressure by face mask, and placement of an oral airway may aid in relieving the obstruction.
- Consider IV induction in patients with severe OSA, since IV induction can rapidly induce a deep plane of anesthesia ready for airway instrumentation.
- Sedative and anesthetic medications alter the CO_2 response curve, theoretically placing OSA patients at higher risk of sedation and anesthesia induced respiratory complications. Sedatives or residual anesthetics may make it impossible for patients to arouse themselves during obstructive episodes. Therefore, short-acting anesthetics should be chosen.
- Excessive doses of opiates may precipitate postoperative hypoventilation and airway obstruction in OSA patients. Careful titration of short-acting opioids is important to avoid airway problems postoperatively.
- Rectal acetaminophen (30-40 mg/kg) can be used as an adjunct for pain management.
- Patients should be awake and have adequate strength to maintain the upper airway before tracheal extubation. Patients with severe OSA and those with comorbidities are at risk of persistent OSA after surgery.
- Efforts should be made to reduce the risk of postoperative vomiting and pain after adenotonsillectomy. Steroids have been shown to improve postoperative oral intake and reduce pain and vomiting. A dosing study of IV dexamethasone for adenotonsillectomy showed that a low dose (0.0625 mg/kg) is just as effective as a high dose (1 mg/kg) in reducing postoperative pain and vomiting. We administer dexamethasone 0.5 mg/kg IV, for a maximum dose of 10 mg IV.
- Administer an antiemetic, as adenotonsillectomy is one of the most emetogenic procedures, with an incidence of vomiting up to 70% when no antiemetic is used.

POSTOPERATIVE CONSIDERATIONS

- Patients with OSA may have decreased sensitivity to CO_2 in the postoperative period and may need ventilator support, as their hypoxic drive to breathe may be abolished by O_2 as well as subanesthetic concentrations of inhaled anesthetics or sedatives.
- Small doses of sedatives, opioids, anesthetics, and muscle relaxants may cause prolonged upper airway muscle relaxation in excess of diaphragmatic relaxation, predisposing the OSA patient to postobstructive desaturation and pulmonary edema after extubation.
- A diagnosis of OSA increases the risk for postoperative respiratory morbidity from 1% to 20%. Careful respiratory monitoring in the immediate postoperative period is important to detect obstruction and consequent postoperative pulmonary edema.
- Postoperative complications include oxygen desaturation <90%, increased work of breathing, and changes on a chest radiograph (edema, atelectasis, infiltrate, pneumothorax, pneumomediastinum, or pleural effusion). Complications associated with severe OSA include laryngospasm, apnea, pulmonary edema, pulmonary hypertensive crisis, pneumonia, and perioperative death.
- The child who continues to have significant obstructive episodes after extubation can be positioned in the lateral decubitus or prone position to help relieve the obstruction. CPAP or BiPAP can be used to assist ventilation and relieve airway collapse. The placement of a nasal airway before extubation might be considered in more severe cases. Reintubation may be required in an occasional patient.
- Before discharge from the recovery room, the oxygen saturation on room air should return to the preoperative baseline value, and the patient should not become hypoxic or develop obstruction when left undisturbed.
- American Society of Anesthesiologists (ASA) practice guidelines suggest that OSA patients should be monitored 3 hours longer than their non-OSA counterparts before discharge. Monitoring should continue for a median of 7 hours (possibly overnight) after the last episode of airway obstruction or hypoxemia while breathing room air in an unstimulated environment.
- ASA practice guidelines recommend admission for children <3 years of age who undergo adenotonsillectomy.
- Consider admission to the intensive care unit (ICU) or a monitored ward in the following patients:

  - Age <24 months
  - Weight >97th percentile or morbid obese
  - Any significant neuromuscular disease (eg, muscular dystrophies, myasthenia, myopathies, spinal cord disorders, mitochondrial and

glycogen storage diseases, severe cerebral palsy that may be associated with central apnea)
- Genetic or chromosomal syndromes prone to airway obstruction (Down syndrome, Pierre Robin syndrome and Treacher Collins syndrome, mucopolysaccharidoses such as Hunter and Hurler syndromes, craniofacial syndromes, achondroplasia)
- Complex or cyanotic congenital heart disease
- Cor pulmonale, right ventricular hypertrophy, or pulmonary hypertension
- Significant hematologic disorders, cogulopathies, or factor deficiencies
- Sickle cell disease
- Previous trauma or burns to the airway, face, or neck
- Postoperative complications include oxygen desaturation <90%, increased work of breathing, and changes on a chest radiograph (edema, atelectasis, infiltrate, pneumothorax, pneumomediastinum, or pleural effusion). Complications associated with severe OSA include laryngospasm, apnea, pulmonary edema, pulmonary hypertensive crisis, pneumonia, and perioperative death.

DOs and DON'Ts

✓   Do try to determine the severity of OSA in patients who have not had polysomnography.
✓   Do use short-acting anesthetics.
✓   Do monitor OSA patients for 3 hours longer than their non-OSA counterparts before discharge.
⊗   Do not give postoperative opioids without appropriate monitoring.
✓   Do reserve an ICU bed for postoperative care of severe OSA patients.
⊗   Do not use the STOP-BANG tool to assess risk for OSA. Only STOP is applicable in the pediatric population.

CONTROVERSIES

Low dose (0.0625 mg/kg) of IV dexamethasone vs high dose (1 mg/kg) in reducing postoperative pain and vomiting.

SURGICAL CONCERNS

Postoperative bleeding is a potentially serious complication following adenotonsillectomy.

FACTOID

Components of polysomnography recommended by the American Thoracic Society:

- Respiratory effort—assessed by abdominal and chest wall movement
- Airflow at nose, mouth, or both
- Arterial oxygen saturation
- End-tidal CO_2 or transcutaneous CO_2 (recommended specifically for pediatric polysomnography to detect hypoventilation)
- Electrocardiograph
- Electromyography (tibial) to monitor arousals
- Electroencephalography, electrooculography, and electromyography for sleep staging

STOP-BANG TOOL

STOP

Snoring: Do you snore loudly (louder than talking or loud enough to be heard through closed doors)?

Tiredness: Do you often feel tired, fatigued, or sleepy during the day?

Observed stopped breathing: Has anyone observed you stop breathing during your sleep?

Blood Pressure: Do you have or are you being treated for high blood pressure?

BANG

BMI >35

Age >50

Neck circumference >40 cm

Gender male

Yes to 3 or more questions = high risk of obstructive sleep apnea.
Yes to less than 3 questions = low risk of obstructive sleep apnea.

In the pediatric population, answering yes to 2 or more questions in the STOP tool places the pediatric patient at a high risk of OSA. Answering no to less than 2 questions places the pediatric patient at a low risk of OSA.

Reference

Chung F, Yegneswaran B, Lia P, et al. STOP questionnaire: A tool to screen patients for obstructive sleep apnea. *Anesthesiology* 2008;108(5):812-821.

3 POSTTONSILLECTOMY BLEEDING

Neeta R. Saraiya, MD

YOUR PATIENT

A 10-year-old female presents to the emergency room with a history of spitting blood-tinged secretions for 2 days and vomiting blood in the last 12 hours. The patient's past surgical history is significant for having had an adenotonsillectomy done 8 days earlier.

Upon examination, patient is sitting in bed, anxious. Vitals: HR 120/min; BP 100/50; respiratory rate 24/min.

Labs: HCT 30%; platelets 220K/µL; INR 1.2.

PREOPERATIVE CONSIDERATIONS

Posttonsillectomy bleeding is a common complication following adeno-tonsillectomy. Bleeding can be primary; this occurs within the first 24 hours after surgery in <1% of the patients. Secondary bleeding occurs between 5 and 12 days after surgery in about 4% of the patients and may be due to sloughing of the eschar from the tonsillar bed, loosening of ties, or infection from underlying chronic tonsillitis.

Most of the blood is swallowed; therefore, it is difficult to estimate the amount of blood loss. The patient may be hypovolemic due to blood loss or have poor oral intake due to pain and bleeding. There may be an underlying coagulopathy that is still undiagnosed at the time of presentation.

There is a potential for difficult intubation because of difficulty in visualizing the larynx secondary to bleeding obscuring the view and edema from the previous surgery. Patients are at risk for pulmonary aspiration because of the presence of large amounts of sequestered intragastric blood at the time of the induction of anesthesia.

ANESTHETIC MANAGEMENT

- Use awake IV placement.
- Use preoxygenation with rapid sequence induction with cricoid pressure with propofol or etomidate and succinylcholine or rocuronium.
- Have two suctions available in case one clots while you are trying to intubate.

- Intubate with an oral Ring-Adair-Elwyn cuffed endotracheal tube.
- Maintain with volatile agents + IV narcotics.
- Intraoperative blood transfusion may be required.
- Once hemostasis is achieved, suction the stomach with a large-bore nasogastric tube.
- Extubate the patient when fully awake and place the patient in a left lateral position.

POSTOPERATIVE CONSIDERATIONS

Patients are monitored in the postanesthesia care unit after extubation for any signs of bleeding or hemodynamic instability and are admitted to the floor postoperatively. They are discharged home when there is no further sign of bleeding, and have resumed eating, drinking, and their pain is well controlled.

DOs and DON'Ts

⊗   Do not try suctioning the stomach prior to induction.
✓   Do place a large-bore IV for hydration and volume resuscitation.
⊗   Do not attempt inhalation induction.
✓   Do send a type and cross for blood and know about blood availability prior to starting the case.

SURGICAL REPAIR

A tonsillectomy can be either partial or total and can be either intracapsular or extracapsular. Different surgical techniques are used to perform tonsillectomy; for example, cold dissection, electrosurgery using a monopolar blade, bipolar, monopolar suction, harmonic scalpel, laser dissection, coblation, and argon plasma coagulation.

FACTOID

Tonsillectomy with or without adenoidectomy is one of the most common surgeries performed, with more than 300,000 tonsillectomies being performed annually. The most common indication for tonsillectomy is a sleep-related breathing disorder (obstructive sleep apnea), followed by recurrent tonsillitis.

4 BILATERAL MYRINGOTOMY AND TUBES IN A PATIENT WITH AN UPPER RESPIRATORY TRACT INFECTION

Neeta R. Saraiya, MD

YOUR PATIENT

An otherwise healthy 2-year-old male child presents with a history of multiple ear infections and hearing loss. He has just completed a course of amoxicillin for a recent ear infection. He has symptoms of a recent acute upper airway infection and still has a runny nose.

PREOPERATIVE CONSIDERATIONS

Otitis media with effusion is the most common chronic condition of the ear in children. Children have small eustachian tubes and are unable to clear the mucus secreted in the mastoid and middle ear. Children with Down syndrome and craniofacial anomalies like cleft palate are more prone to develop middle ear infections. Fluid may also develop in the middle ear during an upper respiratory infection.

Persistent effusion can cause conductive hearing loss and predispose the child to develop recurrent acute suppurative otitis media.

Patients with recent upper respiratory tract infections (URI) are at increased risk for respiratory complications following general anesthesia (desaturations, laryngospasm, or bronchospasm). These can easily be treated with oxygen, positive pressure ventilation, and inhaled bronchodilators. However, some patients may have severe bronchospasm requiring postoperative intubation and intensive care unit admission or postoperative pneumonia. Deciding when to cancel cases is sometimes difficult because of a variety of factors. In general, patients who have only upper airway symptoms, no fever, and no history of pulmonary disease can be taken care of safely, but a discussion should be had with the family and the surgeon evaluating the risks and benefits of proceeding. The risks remain elevated for up to 6 weeks following an acute URI, so the timing of rescheduling a case can also be problematic.

ANESTHETIC MANAGEMENT

- Use mask induction.
- Maintain anesthesia with either a mask or a laryngeal mask airway (LMA).
- It may or may not be necessary to place an IV in a healthy child, since this is a short procedure that may take about 10-15 minutes.
- Intranasal fentanyl 1-2 μg/kg and rectal acetaminophen 30-40 mg/kg; make sure the next dose of acetaminophen will be given no sooner than 6 hours later.
- Nerve block of the auricular branch of the vagus (nerve of Arnold) behind the tragus may be performed with 0.2 mL of 0.25% bupivacaine to manage postoperative pain.

POSTOPERATIVE CONSIDERATIONS

Nearly all patients who have had tube placement have occasional episodes of otorrhea through the tube. Patients are discharged home within 1 to 2 hours after the procedure. Tubes can also extrude prematurely, necessitating repeated insertion. Long-term complications from tube placement include persistent perforation after tube extrusion, which may require operative closure; scarring of the tympanic membrane or middle ear structures; and atrophy of the previously incised area of the tympanic membrane. The risk of cholesteatoma is higher in children who have had tubes placed.

DOs and DON'Ts

✓   Do place an IV if the patient has craniofacial anomalies or a history of difficult mask ventilation.

✓   Do place an IV if an LMA is used for the maintenance of anesthesia.

SURGICAL REPAIR

A small incision is commonly made in the inferior quadrant of the tympanic membrane; the posterior superior quadrant is avoided, since there is a risk of injuring the ossicles. The mucus is suctioned from the ear, and a Silastic tube is placed at the myringotomy site.

FACTOID

Up to one-third of patients who have undergone myringotomy and tube placement have recurrent disease after tube extrusion and require surgical reinsertion of the tube. In these cases, concurrent adenoidectomy is considered.

5 CLEFT LIP AND PALATE REPAIR

Gracie M. Almeida-Chen, MD, MPH

YOUR PATIENT

A 10-month-old female is scheduled for repair of a cleft palate. She had her cleft lip repaired at the age of 6 months without complications. The infant was born full term and has no other medical problems.

PREOPERATIVE CONSIDERATIONS

Cleft lip and cleft palate are among the most common congenital anomalies. They may occur alone, as part of a syndrome (there are more than 300 syndromes associated with facial clefting), or as a component of a sequence (for example, with Pierre Robin syndrome). Clefts of the palate may occur through the same mechanisms as cleft lip or be secondary to an anatomic obstruction preventing the medial fusion of the maxillary processes.

Closure of the cleft palate may result in insufficient tissue for development of the normal length or function of the soft palate and therefore may require a posterior pharyngeal flap. Velopharyngeal (VP) insufficiency is the cause of the hypernasal speech, nasal emission, and nasal turbulence.

There are many techniques for repairing a cleft palate, but all of them include a hard palate procedure and a soft palate (velar) procedure. Palatoplasties are performed with the intention of obtaining VP competence and normal speech and are typically performed before the first year of age.

Pharyngoplasties are performed to treat an incompetent VP sphincter that allows inappropriate escape of nasal air during speech, or hypernasality, defined as VP insufficiency. Pharyngoplasties are often performed as secondary speech procedures after a palatoplasty that failed to result in VP competence.

ANESTHETIC MANAGEMENT

- Most patients with a cleft lip or palate can be induced with a standard inhalational induction or IV induction.
- Airway obstruction can usually be managed with the insertion of an oropharyngeal airway and continuous positive airway pressure.

- For the patient with an isolated cleft lip and palate, difficulty with laryngoscopy is common. Factors predicting a more difficult laryngoscopic view include bilateral clefts and retrognathia. A wide oral opening will help to prevent the laryngoscope blade from slipping into the alveolar ridge defect during laryngoscopy. The view during laryngoscopy is unusual because of the cleft soft and hard palate, but the defect usually allows good visualization of the larynx.
- Cleft patients with associated craniofacial anomalies or retrognathia may be difficult to ventilate or intubate. Adequacy of mask ventilation should be determined. The patient should remain spontaneously ventilating until the trachea is secured with an endotracheal tube.
- Surgical repair of the cleft palate using a laryngeal mask airway (LMA) has been described. However, disruption of a previous cleft palate repair during the placement of an LMA has also been described, suggesting that care should be taken when placing an LMA in a patient with a history of cleft palate repair.
- An oral Ring-Adair-Elwyn preformed tracheal tube is routinely used for the intubation because the preformed bend in the tube facilitates the use of the mouth retractor. Care should be given to securing the tube and protecting it from unintentional extubation.
- For patients having palate surgery, keeping the mean arterial pressure at 50-60 mm Hg may prevent excessive bleeding from the surgical site. This can be achieved by deepening the anesthetic with inhalation agents, opioids (remifentanil), or α_2-agonists (clonidine or dexmedetomidine).
- Throat packs can result in airway obstruction if they are unintentionally left in place, and confirmation of their removal must take place before extubation.
- The adjunct use of regional anesthesia provides analgesia that is better than that provided by incisional infiltration or opioids alone. The bilateral infraorbital nerve block may be used as an adjunct or as the sole analgesic technique for cleft lip repair. The infraorbital nerve is a sensory nerve that is derived from the second maxillary division of the trigeminal nerve and exits from the infraorbital foramen to enter the pterygopalatine fossa. There are two approaches to the infraorbital nerve block: extraoral (percutaneous) and intraoral. For the extraoral approach, locate the infraorbital foramen and insert a 27-gauge needle toward, but not into, the foramen in the lateral direction. The intraoral approach is achieved by advancing a 27-gauge needle along the inner surface of the lip and cephalad to the infraorbital foramen parallel to the maxillary premolar. First palpate the infraorbital foramen and pull the upper lip superiorly to allow room for the needle and syringe. Keep a finger on the infraorbital foramen during the needle advancement to provide accurate measurement of the desired area. A total volume of 0.5-1.5 mL of bupivacaine 0.25%, levobupivacaine 0.25%,

or ropivacaine 0.2% with 1:200,000 epinephrine is injected after negative aspiration for blood.

- The anterior branch of the greater palatine nerve may also be blocked for cleft palate repair. Using a 27-gauge needle, insert the needle approximately 1 cm from the first and second maxillary molars on the hard palate. Palpate with the needle to find the greater palatine foramen, whose depth is usually less than 10 mm. A total volume of 0.3-0.5 mL of local anesthesia is injected after negative aspiration for blood.

POSTOPERATIVE CONSIDERATIONS

Profound tongue, palate, and pharyngeal edema can occur as a result of venous engorgement after the use of the Dingman-Dott mouth retractor in combination with the Trendelenburg position. It is prudent for surgeons to release the retractor repeatedly throughout the procedure to minimize this risk. Patients experiencing respiratory distress postoperatively need to be reintubated. It may take several days for the edema to resolve.

A suture through the tongue that is taped to the cheek can be used to lift the tongue in case of an airway obstruction during the postoperative period.

Postoperative pain management for cleft lip and palate repair should provide analgesia without respiratory depression, nausea, or vomiting. The best solution is a combination of different medications, usually acetaminophen with the occasional addition of an opioid and an adjunct regional technique.

Arm restraints will prevent the infant from reaching the surgical site.

DOs and DON'Ts

✓ Do maintain spontaneous respiration until the trachea has been intubated and lung ventilation confirmed if the cleft lip or cleft palate is associated with craniofacial anomalies or retrognathia.

⊗ Do not use muscle relaxants until the airway is secure and lung ventilation is confirmed in patients with difficult airways.

✓ Do prepare to reintubate if the patient experiences respiratory distress due to airway edema.

CONTROVERSIES

Patients undergoing a palatoplasty who have a history of a difficult airway or have an associated congenital anomaly may have a nasopharyngeal airway placed by the surgeon before emergence. This may help maintain a patent airway and decrease the work of breathing after extubation. However, ischemia from the pressure is a major concern after soft tissue procedures.

A debate on the timing of cleft lip repair exists, especially when it is being done for cosmetic reasons to facilitate parental bonding and social integration.

SURGICAL CONCERNS

Typically, surgical repair of the cleft lip is performed at 3-6 months to ensure adequate feeding, and repair of the cleft palate is performed at 9-18 months to facilitate speech development.

FACTOID

Historically, repair of a cleft lip and palate was performed with no anesthesia. The procedure consisted of reapproximating pared tissue edges. These simple and quick procedures were performed on older children or adults who could tolerate the pain and inconvenience of the procedure.

Cleft lip and palate medical missions are among the most common and are carried out by multiple organizations around the world.

6 EPIGLOTTITIS

Gracie M. Almeida-Chen, MD, MPH

YOUR PATIENT

A 4-year-old female presents to the emergency room with inspiratory stridor, excessive drooling, and substernal retractions and fever. She complains of a sore throat.

PREOPERATIVE CONSIDERATIONS

Epiglottitis begins with a high fever and a sore throat. Other symptoms may include abnormal breathing sounds (stridor), chills and shaking, cyanosis, drooling, dyspnea (the patient may need to sit upright and lean slightly forward in order to breathe), dysphagia, dysphonia, and voice changes (hoarseness). The etiology of epiglottitis is bacterial: *Haemophilus influenzae* type b (75% of cases), Group A β-hemolytic *Streptococcus pneumoniae*, *Staphylococcus aureus*, and *Klebsiella pneumoniae*.

Examination of the upper airway should be limited to noting the respiratory rate, assessing the work of breathing, and observing the level of respiratory distress. No manipulation or examination of the mouth or pharynx should be performed unless it is in a controlled setting. The anesthesiologist must be certain that all necessary broncho-scopes, endotracheal tubes, and emergency tracheostomy equipment are available. A skilled otolaryngologist must be present and should accompany the child at all times once the diagnosis is suspected, should the need for a surgical airway arise.

No blood work should be done, and no intravenous catheter should be placed. The child should be disturbed as little as possible. If parental separation would cause undue anxiety, the parents should be allowed into the operating room.

Concerns regarding a full stomach are theoretically reasonable, as these children have not fasted. However, these children are often so sick, and swallowing is so painful, that food and fluid intake has probably decreased prior to presentation.

ANESTHETIC MANAGEMENT

- Maintain the child in a sitting position and provide general inhalational anesthesia with 100% oxygen and sevoflurane. The ability to transfer gas to allow for oxygenation, removal of CO_2, and the uptake of inhalation agents may be severely restricted by the size of the orifice at the glottic inlet. An inhalational induction with sevoflurane may be quite prolonged as a result of this restricted gas flow.

- Spontaneous ventilation is maintained with gentle assisted respirations as needed until the patient is deep enough to allow for IV placement. Standard American Society of Anesthesiologists monitors are placed.
- Opioids and muscle relaxants are avoided until the airway is established.
- With the child deep and spontaneously ventilating, the otolaryngologist will perform a direct laryngoscopy and rigid bronchoscopy. Visualization of the larynx is often difficult, and the epiglottis needs to be lifted very gently with a blade or a rigid bronchoscope. Because of airway swelling and secretions, an endotracheal tube one to two sizes smaller than would be appropriate for the age and size of the patient is placed.
- If during the induction, any problem leading to a loss of spontaneous ventilation or airway obstruction arises, an emergent direct laryngoscopy or rigid bronchoscopy needs to be attempted.
- The surgeon must be prepared for an emergent cricothyrotomy or tracheostomy if the airway is not quickly achieved.

POSTOPERATIVE CONSIDERATIONS

- Antibiotics and corticosteroids are the mainstays of treatment.
- The patient typically remains sedated with an endotracheal tube in place for at least 24-72 hours.
- Extubation is performed after the resolution of clinical signs and the confirmation of decreased epiglottic swelling by flexible nasal fiberoptic bronchoscopy or direct laryngoscopy in the operating room.

DOs and DON'Ts

✓ Do maintain spontaneous respiration until the trachea has been intubated and lung ventilation confirmed.
✓ Do have a skilled otolaryngologist accompany the child at all times once the diagnosis is suspected, in case the need for a surgical airway should arise.
⊗ Do not manipulate or examine the mouth or pharynx other than in a controlled setting.
⊗ Do not use muscle relaxants until the airway is secure and lung ventilation is confirmed.

CONTROVERSIES

Because of low vaccination rates, the incidence of epiglottitis is increasing.

SURGICAL CONCERNS

The surgeon must be prepared for an emergent cricothyrotomy or tracheostomy if the airway is not achieved quickly.

FACTOID

Until the 1980s, before the Hib vaccine, preschool children between the ages of 2 and 6 years had the highest incidence of epiglottitis, although it also occurred in infants, older children, and occasionally adults.

The classic lateral neck radiographic findings are a swollen epiglottis (ie, a thumb sign), thickened aryepiglottic folds, and obliteration of the vallecula (vallecula sign).

7 POSTOPERATIVE STRIDOR

Gracie M. Almeida-Chen, MD, MPH

YOUR PATIENT

A 4-year-old male status post inguinal hernia repair develops post-operative stridor in the postanesthesia care unit (PACU).

PREOPERATIVE CONSIDERATIONS

Stridor is noisy breathing coupled with increased inspiratory efforts, such as nasal and rib-cage flaring and suprasternal and sternal retraction. Severe airway obstruction may result in cyanosis, respiratory distress and fatigue, pneumothorax, pneumomediastinum, and death. Inspiratory stridor indicates lesions above the vocal cords. Lesions distal to the vocal cords usually produce expiratory stridor. Biphasic stridor is most characteristic of obstruction at the level of the subglottic space.

Postextubation stridor manifests as a barky or croupy cough; it usually develops within the first hour after extubation, but it can develop as late as 24 hours after extubation. It arises from glottic and subglottic edema caused by ischemia of the tracheal mucosa as a result of pressure by the endotracheal tube (ETT). The symptoms appear after extubation because compression by the ETT prevents narrowing of the tracheal lumen. Upon the removal of the ETT, edema develops and narrows the tracheal lumen. Symptoms include expiratory stridor, hoarseness, and chest retractions. If the airway obstruction becomes severe, arterial desaturation occurs, and reintubation may be required to maintain a patent airway.

The following factors increase the risk of postextubation stridor:

- ETT: Tightly fitting in the trachea with a leak pressure above 25 cm H_2O. Leak pressure should be between 10 and 25 cm H_2O to permit ventilation and to maintain perfusion of the tracheal mucosa.
- Age: Children younger than 4 years old are at greater risk because of their disproportionately smaller airway lumen.
- Intubation maneuver: Risk increases with multiple and/or traumatic attempts.
- Duration of endotracheal intubation: Risk for trauma or ischemia increases with prolonged intubation.
- Head or neck surgery: Frequent position changes of the head and neck increase the risk for trauma or ischemia of tracheal mucosa.

- Ongoing upper airway infection or a recent bout of infectious croup: Tracheal mucosa is inflamed and edematous.
- Extubation: Coughing vigorously when an ETT is present.
- Subglottic stenosis: Congenital or acquired lesions or syndromes associated with a disproportionately narrow airway for age, such as Down syndrome.

Intravenous administration of dexamethasone prior to extubation helps to reduce airway swelling if the patient is undergoing airway surgery or has experienced multiple and traumatic attempts at intubation.

ANESTHETIC MANAGEMENT

- Management of postoperative agitation: Crying and agitation in the PACU exacerbates stridor and difficulty in breathing. Sedation and pain control prevent crying and agitation and promote smooth respiration.
- Cool and humidified mist ameliorates postextubation stridor by reducing mucosal edema. It is recommended for mild cases when only stridor is present.
- Racemic epinephrine (dose: 0.05 mL/kg of 2.25% racemic epinephrine [maximum dose 0.5 mL] diluted into 3-5 mL of normal saline, administered by nebulizer over 5-10 minutes) is recommended for moderate postextubation stridor, such as when retractions and dyspnea occur. This reduces mucosal edema via vasoconstriction. The patient should be observed for 4 hours after administration for a potential "rebound effect"—the stridor could recur as the drug's effects dissipate.
- Heliox—a gas that is less dense than air—increases laminar flow and reduces turbulent flow. It works temporarily to alleviate symptoms of upper airway obstruction and prevent the need for reintubation until other therapies become effective or the disease process resolves naturally.
- Corticosteroids decrease airway swelling by interrupting inflammation resulting from intubation-induced airway injury. Dexamethasone dose: 0.5 mg/kg every 4-6 hours, for a maximum of 40 mg/day for 2 days in patients at high risk before extubation.
- In patients with severe stridor and impending respiratory failure that is unresponsive to these treatments, reintubation should be performed before postobstructive pulmonary edema, hypoxemia, and acidosis ensue. An ETT 0.5 mm smaller than predicted should be used, with the size confirmed by the leak test. The ETT should be left in place for 24-48 hours to allow the swelling to subside. Sedation should be provided to avoid further airway trauma.

POSTOPERATIVE CONSIDERATIONS

The decision to discharge a patient home depends on the severity of the symptoms and their clinical course.

- In mild cases (inspiratory stridor with minimal agitation where cool mist, sedation, and pain management are sufficient), patients may be discharged after surgery if the stridor is resolving and has not worsened after an extra hour of observation.
- For moderate cases (stridor, moderate dyspnea, and suprasternal retractions during inspiration, where nebulized racemic epinephrine and dexamethasone are added to the treatment), patients may be discharged home after the symptoms have improved and the window for a potential rebound effect from racemic epinephrine has passed with no further stridor. Patients should be admitted if symptoms are not improving significantly and additional doses of nebulized racemic epinephrine are administrated, especially in infants.
- For severe cases (stridor with severe difficulty breathing, intercostal retractions, inability to maintain oxygenation, lethargy), patients should be reintubated with a smaller ETT and admitted to the pediatric intensive care unit.

DOs and DON'Ts

✓ Do maintain air leak around ETT <25 cm H_2O.
✓ Do delay elective surgery if intubation is required in a child with an upper respiratory infection.
⊗ Do not allow patients to cough vigorously prior to extubation.
⊗ Do not perform multiple attempts at intubation or traumatic intubation.
✓ Do administer dexamethasone in patients undergoing airway surgery and in patients who have experienced multiple and/or traumatic attempts at intubation.
✓ Do reintubate with a smaller ETT in patients with severe stridor.

SURGICAL CONCERNS

The surgeon must be prepared for an emergent cricothyrotomy or tracheostomy if the airway is so edematous that an intubation is not possible in patients with severe stridor.

FACTOID

Stridor in pediatric patients may be congenital or acquired. Most cases are of extrathoracic origin, but some originate in the large intrathoracic airways (trachea or major bronchi).

8 SUBGLOTTIC STENOSIS

Gracie M. Almeida-Chen, MD, MPH

YOUR PATIENT

A 4-year-old male with congenital subglottic stenosis and a tracheotomy presents for laryngotracheal reconstruction. He has inspiratory and expiratory stridor that is always present.

PREOPERATIVE CONSIDERATIONS

Congenital subglottic stenosis results from embryologic failure that includes laryngeal atresia, stenosis, and webs. In its mildest form, congenital subglottic stenosis shows a normal-appearing cricoid with a smaller-than-average diameter, usually with an elliptical shape. Infants and children with mild subglottic stenosis may present with a history of recurrent upper respiratory infections, often diagnosed as croup, in which minimal glottic swelling precipitates airway obstruction. The location of the stenosis is usually 2-3 mm below the true vocal cords.

Severe congenital subglottic stenosis can be a life-threatening airway emergency that manifests immediately after the infant is delivered. Tracheotomy at the time of delivery can be lifesaving.

Neonatal subglottic stenosis that is unresponsive to nonoperative therapy may require tracheotomy or an anterior cricoid split procedure. After tracheotomy and without an endotracheal tube to act as a stent, the stenosis may become more severe. Over the next few years, the airway may heal, allowing for decannulation, but laryngotracheal reconstructive (LTR) surgery may be necessary to allow for decannulation.

The five stages of laryngotracheal reconstruction are characterization of the stenosis, expansion of the tracheal lumen, stabilization of the framework, healing of the airway, and decannulation.

An anterior cartilage graft with a tracheotomy left in place without a stent is indicated primarily for an isolated anterior subglottic stenosis with no or relatively mild posterior subglottic components. A variation of this procedure is to remove the tracheotomy at the time of surgery and perform a single-stage laryngotracheoplasty. Posterior division of the cricoid plate and the introduction of a cartilage graft between the cut ends are indicated particularly for children with persistent posterior glottic pathology or primarily posterior subglottic pathology.

Single-stage LTR uses cartilage grafts to provide stability for the reconstructed airway. Single-stage LTR may include an anterior cartilage graft, a posterior cartilage graft, or both, and reconstruction often includes a cartilage graft at the former stoma site. The grafts are supported temporarily by a full-length endotracheal tube fixed in position through the nasal route. Children usually remain intubated for 7-10 days for anterior cartilage grafts alone, and for 12-14 days if a posterior and anterior graft is required.

ANESTHETIC MANAGEMENT

The patient may be anesthetized by the intravenous route or with inhalation anesthesia through a tracheotomy cannula. The patient is placed in the tracheotomy position with the shoulders elevated and the neck hyperextended. A tracheotomy tube is replaced with a sterile cuffed armored (anode) endotracheal tube through the tracheostomy stoma and is covered under an adhesive drape to minimize contamination of the surgical field.

An auricular or septal rib cartilage is used for grafting. Toward the conclusion of surgery, the armored tube is removed from the tracheostomy stoma and replaced with a cuffed oral endotracheal tube (ETT) or nasotracheal tube, one size larger than is appropriate for the patient's age and size, to stent the larynx. This intraoperative transition needs to be carefully coordinated between the anesthesiologist and the surgeon.

POSTOPERATIVE CONSIDERATIONS

- Children usually remain intubated for 7-10 days for anterior cartilage grafts alone, and for 12-14 days if a posterior and anterior graft is required.
- One requirement for single-stage laryngotracheal reconstruction is meticulous postoperative management of the patient's condition in the intensive care unit (ICU). The oral ETT or nasotracheal airway must be maintained securely during the time of extended stenting without accidental extubation.
- Some centers use sedation to prevent agitation and accidental self-extubation and to avoid pharmacologic paralysis. However, many children do not tolerate intubation and require prolonged sedation and neuromuscular blockade to ensure maintenance of an airway with minimal trauma during healing. If neuromuscular blockade is used, daily recovery of neuromuscular function and the avoidance of prolonged use of corticosteroids will be associated with less muscle weakness after extubation.
- Prolonged sedation with benzodiazepines or opioids can lead to withdrawal syndrome, and close observation after weaning from these

agents is important. The use of dexmedetomidine in pediatric patients for prolonged sedation in the ICU should be considered.

- Postoperative antibiotics, antireflux medications, and dexamethasone may be required.

DOs and DON'Ts

✓ Do listen for stridor. Subglottic stridor is usually biphasic in nature because the structures are rigid, and no collapse of tissue occurs during either phase of respiration. It is a fixed obstruction.

✓ Do document the timing, onset, and duration of stridor, voice or cry quality, feeding abnormalities or failure to thrive, cyanosis, recurrent croup, or hospitalizations for respiratory illnesses and possible foreign body aspiration.

✓ Do perform a physical exam that includes a thorough head and neck exam, as well as careful characterization of stridor and signs of respiratory distress.

✓ Do have an ear, nose, and throat surgeon perform a flexible laryngoscopic exam. An assessment of laryngomalacia, vocal cord paralysis, laryngopharyngeal reflux, or other laryngeal pathology should be documented.

⊗ Do not use high peak airway pressures—this creates an increased risk of suture dehiscence.

⊗ Do not allow patients to become agitated in the ICU and self-extubate.

CONTROVERSIES

Controversy exists over the use of neuromuscular blockade in the ICU to ensure maintenance of an airway with minimal trauma during healing.

SURGICAL CONCERNS

Complications of laryngotracheal reconstruction include bleeding, pneumothorax, pneumomediastinum, recurrent laryngeal nerve injury, slipped graft, slipped stent, plugged stent, wound infection, keloid formation, suprastomal or infrastomal collapse, restenosis, tracheocutaneous fistula, granulation tissue, and death.

FACTOID

The Myer-Cotton staging system is useful for mature, firm, circumferential subglottic stenosis. It describes the stenosis based on the percent relative

TABLE 8-1   PERCENTAGE (%) OBSTRUCTION ESTIMATED BY ENDOTRACHEAL TUBE SIZE

Age of Patient	ID 2.0*	ID 2.5	ID 3.0	ID 3.5	ID 4.0	ID 4.5	ID 5.0	ID 5.5
Premature	40	—	—	—	—	—	—	—
	58	30	—	—	—	—	—	—
0-3 months	68	48	26	—	—	—	—	—
3-9 months	75	59	41	22	—	—	—	—
9 months to 2 years	80	67	53	38	20	—	—	—
2 years	84	74	62	50	35	19	—	—
4 years	86	78	68	57	45	32	17	—
6 years	89	81	73	64	54	43	30	16

*ID = Internal diameter of the endotracheal tube. Endotracheal tube size is used for characterizing firm, mature subglottic stenosis. The size is determined by placement of an endotracheal tube that leaks at 10-25 cm H_2O. The numbers in the columns indicate the percentage of obstruction.

reduction in cross-sectional area of the subglottis, which is determined by differing sized endotracheal tubes (Table 8-1).

Children with less than 70% obstruction usually do not require surgical intervention. However, children with these conditions may have intermittent airway symptoms, especially when infection or inflammation causes mucosal edema.

9 CYSTIC HYGROMA

Susan Y. Lei, MD

YOUR PATIENT

A healthy 6-month-old female with recent upper respiratory infection who has been found to have a cystic hygroma presents for magnetic resonance imaging to determine the extent of the lesion. She developed stridor after her respiratory infection.

> *Neck x-ray*: Large soft tissue growth in left lateral neck with mild tracheal deviation, trachea patent.
> *Physical exam*: 7 kg. Large, mobile, bluish soft tissue bulge in lateral neck. Inspiratory stridor 99% O_2 saturation on room air.

PREOPERATIVE CONSIDERATIONS

Cystic hygroma, also known as cystic lymphangioma, is a benign congenital malformation of the lymphatic system that typically affects the head and neck (75% of the time) with a left predilection, the axilla (20% of the time), and, more infrequently, the mediastinum, groin, and retroperitoneum. It is a result of a failure of the lymphatics to connect to the venous system, abnormal budding of the lymphatic tissue, and sequestered lymphatic rests that retain their embryonic growth potential, resulting in penetration of adjacent structures and fascial planes leading to retention of secretions as a result of a lack of venous drainage.

The incidence of cystic hygromas is 1:12,000 births. More than 50% of cystic hygromas are present at birth, with 80-90% presenting by age 2. Some people believe that all cystic hygromas are present at birth but are undetected. They can be visualized prenatally with ultrasound by 10 weeks' gestation. They often present after a sudden increase in size as a result of an upper respiratory infection or intralesional bleeding. Spontaneous shrinkage or decompression of a cystic hygroma is uncommon. Giant cystic hygromas can involve both sides of the face and neck and extend to the mediastinum, causing acute airway obstruction and compression of the main vessels.

Genetic abnormalities are present in 25-75% of children with cystic hygroma. They are commonly found in Turner syndrome, Down syndrome, Klinefelter syndrome, trisomy 18, and trisomy 13. In addition, intrauterine alcohol exposure has been associated with cystic hygroma formation.

When cystic hygroma is suspected prenatally, patients should undergo chromosomal analysis or amniocentesis. Magnetic resonance imaging is the gold standard test to delineate the composition, location, and extent of the lesion. Careful observation of the cystic hygroma is recommended for asymptomatic patients only, and while medical treatment with sclerosing agents is available, the definitive treatment is still surgical excision in one- or multistage resections.

A thorough preoperative history and physical examination focusing on signs and symptoms of airway compression, respiratory distress, cough, stridor, tachypnea, dysphagia, and dyspnea are important. Carefully review imaging studies such as x-ray, CT scan, and MRI of the chest and neck to assess the size, position, and extent of the tumor. It is important to note the position of the tongue relative to the mass, as this can impede visualization during direct laryngoscopy. Also note the vascularity of the lesion.

On physical exam, palpate the trachea to rule out deviation and assess respiratory status in different positions to assess for compression of mediastinal structures.

ANESTHETIC MANAGEMENT

- Consider premedication with anticholinergic drugs such as glycopyrrolate or atropine to decrease oral secretions. Use caution with anxiolytic agents, as these can lead to sedation and hypoventilation, which can further exacerbate airway obstruction.
- Different size endotracheal tubes, laryngeal mask airways (LMAs), nasal airways, and oral airways should be available, along with different blades for intubation. Have difficult airway equipment and a fiberoptic scope ready in the room. An ear, nose, and throat surgeon should be present on standby and ready to perform a tracheotomy if necessary.
- IV placement should take place prior to induction.
- If the tumor involves the tongue and oropharyngeal structures, direct laryngoscopy will be very difficult, if not impossible.
- Use awake intubation or intubation with sedation using IV ketamine and midazolam and topical anesthesia. An oral airway or an LMA split lengthwise can be used to assist fiberoptic intubation.
- Mask induction with sevoflurane while maintaining spontaneous ventilation may be attempted if there is no distortion of the tongue or expansion of the lesion into the oropharynx.
- Emergency tracheotomy may be extremely difficult due to distortion of the neck structures and the presence of considerable amounts of lymphatic drainage. Consider aspiration of the cyst if acute airway obstruction develops.

- Maintain anesthesia with sevoflurane.
- Keep the patient intubated until airway edema resolves and there is no evidence of wound hemorrhage.

POSTOPERATIVE CONSIDERATIONS

Patients should be extubated awake in the operating room, with equipment and endotracheal tubes ready for reintubation if the patient obstructs after extubation. Dexamethasone and a racemic epinephrine nebulizer can help reduce supraglottic edema.

DOs and DON'Ts

✓ Do maintain spontaneous ventilation until the airway is secured.
✓ Do have multiple plans for intubation and make preparations in case the airway is lost.
⊗ Do avoid repeated attempts of direct laryngoscopy.
⊗ Do not give opioids prior to intubation.

CONTROVERSIES

- Awake vs asleep intubation.

SURGICAL CONCERNS

Complete resection has been possible in only about 40% of cases. Multistage excisions are more difficult, as they are complicated by fibrosis and distorted anatomical landmarks. Cystic hygromas are benign lesions. If the infant is very small in size and neurovascular structures are involved, it is best to delay surgery until the infant is older if there is no airway obstruction so that structures can be easily identified and visualized.

FACTOID

Cystic hygromas with airway obstruction diagnosed prenatally will require a cesarean delivery and an ex utero intrapartum treatment procedure to secure the airway.

10 ASPIRATED FOREIGN BODY

Neeta R. Saraiya, MD

YOUR PATIENT

A 2-year-old child is brought to the ER. The mother states that an older sibling was eating peanuts and the child grabbed some and put them in his mouth, and since then the child has been irritable and coughing continuously.

Upon exam, the child is coughing with no evidence of acute respiratory distress. There are decreased breath sounds on the right side.

Chest x-ray shows hyperinflation of the right lung.

PREOPERATIVE CONSIDERATIONS

Pediatric airway foreign body aspiration has a high rate of airway distress, morbidity, and mortality in children less than 3 years of age. The peak age for aspiration events is 1-2 years; this is due to incomplete dentition, immature swallowing coordination, and a tendency to be easily distracted while eating. The most common foreign body retrieved is peanuts. Other aspirated items include pieces of food, such as carrots, nuts, candies, grapes, seeds, popcorn, and hot dogs. Nonfood objects include coins, pills, safety pins, marbles, ball bearings, and beads. Food items like nuts can expand and become friable, and, as a result, they get fragmented during their removal and cause further obstruction. Peanuts can release oils and cause chemical irritation. Presenting symptoms vary from no apparent distress to impending respiratory failure, depending on the size and location of the foreign body. Children may also present with coughing, wheezing, shortness of breath, fever, or recurrent pneumonia.

ANESTHETIC MANAGEMENT

- Use mask induction with sevoflurane or IV induction with propofol with spontaneous ventilation.
- IV atropine or glycopyrrolate is given to dry secretions and prevent vagal-induced bradycardia from the insertion of the bronchoscope.
- Maintain anesthesia with total intravenous anesthesia with propofol and/or remifentanil infusion.
- Spray the larynx with 1-2% lidocaine prior to passage of the bronchoscope.

- Use a precordial stethoscope to detect changes in breath sounds or regional ventilation.
- Remain in constant communication with the surgeon.

POSTOPERATIVE CONSIDERATIONS

Patients are placed in a head-up position and monitored for possibility of airway obstruction secondary to edema. If the patient has stridor, humidified oxygen, IV dexamethasone (maximum 10 mg/kg), and nebulized racemic epinephrine (2.25%) (0.05 mL/kg, max 0.5 mL) may be administered. Patients are admitted to the floor or the intensive care unit depending on the degree of lung irritation. They may be discharged home the next day if stable.

DOs and DON'Ts

✓ Do maintain spontaneous ventilation.
⊗ Do not use nitrous oxide, as it can cause air trapping distal to the obstruction.
✓ Do have instruments for emergency cricothyrotomy or tracheotomy available if complete airway obstruction occurs after induction.
⊗ Do not use jet ventilation due to the risk of barotrauma and pneumothorax.

SURGICAL MANAGEMENT

A rigid ventilating bronchoscope with an optical telescope forceps is most commonly used for foreign body removal. The anesthesia circuit is connected to the side arm of the bronchoscope for oxygen delivery and positive pressure ventilation if necessary. Once the foreign body is visualized, it is grasped and an attempt is made to remove it in one piece. The bronchoscope, bronchoscope forceps, and foreign body are removed together to prevent dislodging the foreign body and causing further obstruction. If the foreign body obstructs the subglottis or trachea during extraction, it must be pushed distally into a bronchus to allow ventilation.

FACTOID

In the United States, approximately 150 children die each year from foreign body aspiration. Overall, 95% of the foreign bodies lodge in the right mainstem bronchus, and 5% lodge in the trachea. The foreign bodies are radiolucent 90% of the time, and air trapping, infiltrate, and atelectasis are seen on chest x-ray.

11 LARYNGEAL PAPILLOMATOSIS

Neeta R. Saraiya, MD

YOUR PATIENT

A 7-year-old female patient presents with hoarseness and stridor. The patient has a history of laryngeal papilloma.

PREOPERATIVE CONSIDERATIONS

Laryngeal papillomas are benign epithelial tumors that are caused by infection with the human papillomavirus (HPV). Papillomas can occur at any age; they occur frequently in children under 10 years of age, but in many cases they disappear after the patient has reached adolescence. They most commonly affect the larynx and upper respiratory tract of children, resulting in hoarseness, stridor, obstruction of the airway, and asphyxiation if left untreated. The leading cause of HPV infection in children is infection from the birth canal or the blood of the infected mother.

Papillomas often recur and can spread to the hypolaryngeal vestibules, the epiglottis, and occasionally the trachea and lungs; this may also lead to head and neck cancers. Because of the growth of the papillomas in the narrow pediatric airway, severe laryngeal obstruction may occur. Many children are treated as outpatients and require numerous procedures throughout their childhood to remove the tumors once or twice a month as they reappear. Some children with severe airway obstruction may even need a tracheotomy.

ANESTHETIC MANAGEMENT

- Maintain a patent airway during surgery to ensure adequate ventilation and surgical exposure.
- Use mask or IV induction with propofol with spontaneous ventilation.
- Spray the larynx with 1-2% lidocaine prior to suspension.
- Maintain anesthesia with total intravenous anesthesia with propofol and remifentanil infusion.
- If intubation is needed, a small-size tube is generally used.
- If jet ventilation is needed, then subglottic jet ventilation is used at 20-25 breaths per minute at a pressure starting at 5-10 psi and titrated up while observing chest excursion and oxygen saturation.

POSTOPERATIVE CONSIDERATIONS

Bleeding and edema are typically minimal after surgery, and obstructive symptoms often show immediate improvement. Patients may require humidified oxygen in the postanesthesia care unit. Nebulized racemic epinephrine (2.25%) (0.05 mL/kg, max 0.5 mL) may be administered if patients have stridor. Patients are generally discharged home the day after surgery.

DOs and DON'Ts

⊗   Do not premedicate if the patient has stridor or hoarseness with airway obstruction.
✓   Do maintain spontaneous ventilation.
✓   Do have instruments for emergency cricothyrotomy or tracheotomy available if complete airway obstruction occurs after induction.

SURGICAL REPAIR

Surgical excision of tumors at frequent intervals to relieve the symptoms of airway obstruction is the mainstay of therapy in these patients. Carbon dioxide laser has been used for the excision of laryngeal papillomas. More recently, a laryngeal microdebrider has become the preferred method for excision of the papillomas in many centers.

FACTOID

Human papillomavirus subtypes 6, 11, 16, and 18 have been identified. Although with the availability of human papillomavirus vaccinations, intralesional cidofovir and propranolol may serve as new adjunctive treatments in children with aggressive recurrent respiratory papillomatosis, there are no specific and effective treatments for recurrent pediatric laryngeal papillomatosis.

12 DIFFICULT AIRWAY MANAGEMENT

Philipp J. Houck, MD

YOUR PATIENT

You are called to another operating room by your colleague for a failed intubation on a 2-year-old patient.

PREOPERATIVE CONSIDERATIONS

Most nonsyndromic children are easy to intubate. Typically, "what you see is what you get" is true. Any dysmorphic child, especially those with hypoplastic mandibles or low-set ears, should raise a red flag, and some diseases warrant special mention.

> *Treacher Collins syndrome.* There is an unfortunate combination of difficult mask ventilation and difficult intubation. The difficult mask ventilation is worse than expected from just the physical appearance. Intubation does not get easier with age.
>
> *Pierre-Robin sequence.* Intubation is difficult, but does get better with age. As the mandible grows or is surgically advanced, the intubation gets easier.

Lower airway problems such as anterior mediastinal mass and tracheoesophageal fistula are discussed in the appropriate chapters.

ANESTHETIC MANAGEMENT

- Consider an awake fiberoptic intubation whenever this is a realistic option.
- If an awake fiberoptic intubation is not possible, establish an intravenous access, and consider giving glycopyrrolate 4 μg/kg before inducing anesthesia.
- Inhalational induction of anesthesia is more gradual and is preferred by some anesthesiologists because it is easier to maintain spontaneous ventilation. Induction with propofol might produce a less obstructed airway.
- A regular oral airway can be cut longitudinally and be used as a conduit, similar to the way one would use an Ovassapian or Williams airway in an adult.

- In smaller patients, consider placing a laryngeal mask airway (LMA) before attempting the fiberoptic intubation, then use the LMA as a conduit. Often this will make the fiberoptic intubation easier. Always ensure that the endotracheal tube (ETT) you are planning to use fits through the appropriate LMA size. In some cases, the pilot balloon does not fit through the LMA; in such cases, either the LMA can be left outside the patient or the pilot balloon can be positioned outside the LMA by retrogradely inserting the ETT through the LMA and leaving the pilot balloon in the oropharynx during the use of the LMA. Air-Q LMAs have a removable connector and are designed with fiberoptic intubation in mind.

  The risk of this approach is that if the glottis does not come into view, the LMA has to be removed, and more secretions or blood may make the fiberoptic visualization even harder. Special care must be taken to remove the LMA without removing the endotracheal tube: a long grasper (typically used for direct laryngoscopies by an ear, nose, and throat surgeon) is used to hold the ETT in place as the LMA is removed. Alternatively, a second ETT of the same size can be inserted into the first ETT to make it longer and easier to grasp.

- Do not attempt a direct laryngoscopy for an intubation that is expected to be truly difficult. Use whatever technique is most likely to work on the first attempt. Most anesthesiologists are considering this to be a case for a fiberoptic intubation (Fig. 12-1).

- Fiberoptic intubation and the advancement of the ETT over the fiberoptic scope are easiest in a patient with relaxed vocal cords. Consider paralyzing the patient if you are sure about your ability to mask ventilate.

- Video laryngoscopes are now available in a wide range of variations and sizes. Often the pediatric sizes are simply miniaturized versions. Your experience with a given device is the most important predictor of success.

- After successful intubation, perform a direct laryngoscopy to verifiy that visualization of the larynx is really difficult. This is important information for extubation planning and for the next anesthetic.

POSTOPERATIVE CONSIDERATIONS

Patients who were difficult to ventilate should be not be extubated in the intensive care unit, but should be brought to the operating room for the extubation. Give dexamethasone 0.5 mg/kg (maximum 10 mg) to avoid airway edema after multiple intubation attempts.

Proposal for the management of the unexpected difficult pediatric airway

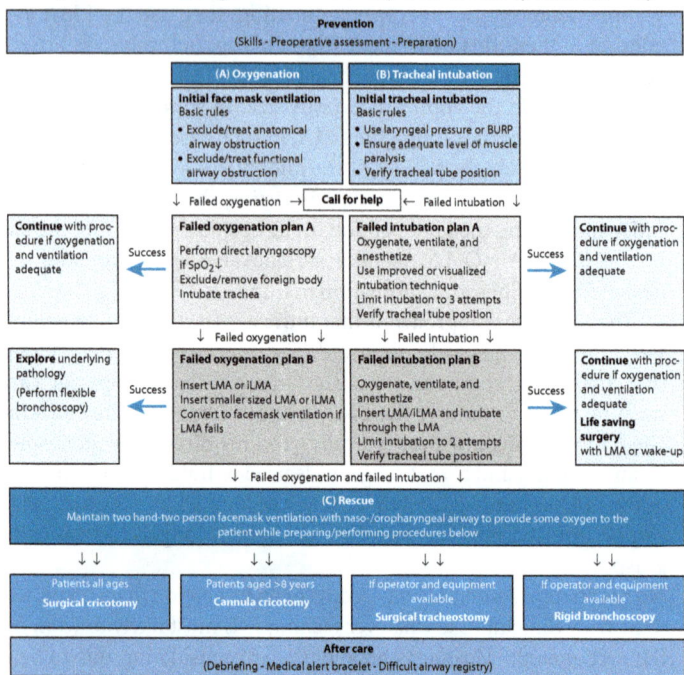

Prevention
(Skills - Preoperative assessment - Preparation)

(A) Oxygenation | **(B) Tracheal intubation**

Initial face mask ventilation
Basic rules
• Exclude/treat anatomical airway obstruction
• Exclude/treat functional airway obstruction

Initial tracheal intubation
Basic rules
• Use laryngeal pressure or BURP
• Ensure adequate level of muscle paralysis
• Verify tracheal tube position

↓ Failed oxygenation → **Call for help** ← Failed intubation ↓

Continue with procedure if oxygenation and ventilation adequate

Failed oxygenation plan A
Perform direct laryngoscopy if SpO₂↓
Exclude/remove foreign body
Intubate trachea
— Success —

Failed intubation plan A
Oxygenate, ventilate, and anesthetize
Use improved or visualized intubation technique
Limit intubation to 3 attempts
Verify tracheal tube position
— Success —

Continue with procedure if oxygenation and ventilation adequate

↓ Failed oxygenation ↓ | ↓ Failed intubation ↓

Explore underlying pathology
(Perform flexible bronchoscopy)
— Success —

Failed oxygenation plan B
Insert LMA or iLMA
Insert smaller sized LMA or iLMA
Convert to facemask ventilation if LMA fails

Failed intubation plan B
Oxygenate, ventilate, and anesthetize
Insert LMA/iLMA and intubate through the LMA
Limit intubation to 2 attempts
Verify tracheal tube position
— Success —

Continue with procedure if oxygenation and ventilation adequate
Life saving surgery with LMA or wake-up

↓ Failed oxygenation and failed intubation ↓

(C) Rescue
Maintain two hand-two person facemask ventilation with naso-/oropharyngeal airway to provide some oxygen to the patient while preparing/performing procedures below

↓↓ | ↓↓ | ↓↓ | ↓↓

Patients all ages
Surgical cricotomy

Patients aged >8 years
Cannula cricotomy

If operator and equipment available
Surgical tracheostomy

If operator and equipment available
Rigid bronchoscopy

After care
(Debriefing - Medical alert bracelet - Difficult airway registry)

FIGURE 12-1 Unanticipated difficult pediatric airway algorithm consisting of three parts: oxygenation, tracheal intubation, and rescue. [Used with permission from Weiss M, Engelhardt T. Proposal for the management of the unexpected difficult pediatric airway, *Pediatric Anesthesia*, 2010;20(5):454-464.]

DOs and DON'Ts

✓ Use only tools that you are experienced with. Practice your skills on elective cases.

✓ Physically verify the compatibility of different sizes of fiberoptic scopes, ETTs, and LMAs prior to using them.

⊗ In cases where you expect difficult ventilation, do not do an inhalational induction without first establishing intravenous access.

✓ Do maintain spontaneous ventilation if you are unsure about the ease of mask ventilation.

✓ Minimal equipment for a difficult intubation is an LMA and a fiberoptic bronchoscope.

⊗ Do not rely on a surgical rescue airway. Minimum age for a cannula cricothyroidotomy is 8 years; surgical airways are time consuming and difficult in smaller children.

CONTROVERSIES

Using muscle relaxants for a difficult intubation is controversial; loss of pharyngeal tone and the complete dependence on positive pressure ventilation are disadvantages. Even most adults with an adequate depth of anesthesia will be unable to recover from a lost airway, regardless of the use of muscle relaxants. It cannot be expected that a small child will recover fast enough to avoid hypoxemia, given the higher oxygen demand and smaller functional residual capacity. Giving muscle relaxants early will avoid functional airway obstruction such as laryngospasm or movement due to inadequate depth of anesthesia ("bucking").

SURGICAL CONCERNS

Patients who are difficult to intubate and ventilate and who need to undergo a series of operations, such as patients with Treacher Collins syndrome, often receive a tracheostomy for safer management.

PART 2

CARDIOVASCULAR

13 CARDIOPULMONARY BYPASS

Riva R. Ko, MD

YOUR PATIENT

A 3-year-old, 13-kg male with a history of an atrial septal defect (ASD) presents for surgical repair with cardiopulmonary bypass (CPB). The patient is asymptomatic and is otherwise healthy.

> *Physical exam*: II/VI systolic murmur, fixed split second heart sound
> *ECG*: Right axis deviation, prolonged PR interval
> *Echocardiogram*: Large ostium secundum ASD

PREOPERATIVE CONSIDERATIONS

An ASD is a common congenital cardiac lesion that requires surgical repair with CPB if it is large. CPB is managed differently in children from the way it is managed in adults because of their different physiology, and it can have different physiologic consequences. The patient's age and the specific lesion, as well as the planned surgical repair, dictate many of the principles of CPB management in children. Some notable differences include:

1. *Priming solution*: Whole blood or packed red blood cells (PRBCs), fresh frozen plasma, and heparin for neonates and infants; PRBCs, crystalloid, albumin, and heparin for children 10-15 kg; crystalloid and heparin for children >15 kg.
2. *Priming volume*: May exceed the blood volume of neonates and infants by 100-200%; more marked effects of hemodilution (eg, decreased hematocrit, reduction in drug levels, coagulopathy).
3. *Pump flow rates*: Wide variation in pediatric patients, from 100-200 mL/kg/min (higher metabolic rate and oxygen demand) to 25-50 mL/kg/min (deep hypothermia).
4. *Perfusion pressure*: 20-50 mm Hg in infants and young children versus 50-80 mm Hg in adults.
5. *Temperature*: Frequent use of deep hypothermic circulatory arrest in pediatric patients (15-20 degrees).

6. *Glucose*: Can have hyperglycemia on CPB from addition of blood products to priming solution, and/or from pre-CPB IV steroid administration; hypoglycemia may also be seen in neonates and infants.
7. *Cannulation*: Increased likelihood of venous obstruction from venous cannula insertion; aortic cannulation complicated by frequent presence of aortopulmonary collaterals, patent ductus arteriosus, and aortic arch abnormalities.

Although surgical repair of an uncomplicated ASD tends to be uneventful and amenable to extubation in the operating room (OR), preoperative discussion with the parents should include the possibility of invasive line placement (and associated complications), postoperative intubation, transfusion of exogenous blood products, neurologic injury, dysrhythmias, need for postoperative pressors and/or pacing, and even death. Premedication with oral midazolam is warranted in anxious children. Lines can be placed after inhalational induction of general anesthesia (GA).

ANESTHETIC MANAGEMENT

- Oral midazolam premedication as needed for anxiety, with or without parental presence in the OR. GA usually is induced via inhalation induction.
- Tailor anesthetic for possible extubation in the OR.
- Arterial line for assessment of blood pressure (BP) on CPB (nonpulsatile flow) and for measurement of activated clotting time (ACT), arterial blood gases (ABGs), hematocrit, and electrolytes. The arterial line generally is placed after induction of GA.
- Either a central venous pressure (CVP) line placed percutaneously (internal jugular [IJ], subclavian, or femoral), or direct transthoracic lines placed by surgeon. For straightforward, uncomplicated ASD repair, CVP may not be necessary in the setting of adequate peripheral IV access.
- Intraoperative transesophageal echocardiography (TEE) (placed prior to incision) to delineate anatomy, adequacy of cardiac de-airing, and ASD repair.
- Two temperature probes, frequently rectal and esophageal or nasopharyngeal.
- Foley catheter for measurement of pre-CPB, CPB, and post-CPB urine output.
- Administer adequate analgesia and muscle relaxation prior to sternotomy; hold ventilation during sternotomy.

- Administer IV heparin 300 units/kg through central line (if there is one) or large-bore peripheral intravenous line; alternatively, the surgeon may inject heparin directly into the heart. Draw arterial blood sample to check ACT prior to initiation of CPB.
- Make sure BP is not elevated prior to aortic cannulation.
- Check patient's head for signs of venous distention after superior vena cava cannulation; consider neurologic monitoring, eg, near-infrared cerebral oximetry or transcranial Doppler. Check with perfusionist regarding adequacy of venous return; ensure lack of large difference between upper and lower body temperatures with cooling (this also may signify a problem with aortic cannula placement).
- Core temperature usually is allowed to drift down for straightforward ASD (ie, no active warming).
- May need vasoactive medications (eg, phenylephrine) to raise perfusion pressure with initiation of CPB.
- Perfusionist will use isoflurane on CPB; consider supplementation with fentanyl, rocuronium, and/or midazolam with rewarming.
- Consider Trendelenburg position after removal of aortic cross-clamp to aid in de-airing the heart.
- Prepare for possible need for pressors post-CPB.
- Ventricular dysrhythmias are commonly seen with unclamping and rewarming; may be transient or require defibrillation and/or medications, eg, lidocaine or magnesium.
- Confirm acceptable ABG and electrolytes with perfusionist prior to separation from CPB.
- Protamine 1-1.3 mg/100 units of original heparin dose once adequacy of repair is confirmed (TEE, hemodynamics); check ACT for assessment of heparin reversal.
- Transfuse as necessary to maximize oxygen delivery and reverse coagulopathy. If transfusion requirements persist despite large amounts of products, consider surgical source of bleeding.

POSTOPERATIVE CONSIDERATIONS

Patients who have undergone a straightforward ASD repair normally are extubated either in the OR or shortly after arrival in the intensive care unit (ICU). Even if extubated, patients will need close monitoring of respiratory status, with particular concern for perioperative complications such as pneumothorax, hemothorax, and atelectasis. The ICU team must be vigilant for common postoperative complications such as bleeding and dysrhythmias. Volume replacement may be necessary to treat hypovolemia-induced low cardiac output; alternatively, some diuresis may be required initially due to increased fluid retention caused by CPB.

DOs and DON'Ts

✓   Do place an arterial catheter either before or after induction of GA. Radial artery cannulation is preferred.

⊗   Do not administer overly high doses of narcotic if planning for early extubation.

✓   Do use intraoperative TEE; consider central line placement.

✓   Do use two temperature probes to measure core temperature (eg, rectal and esophageal).

✓   Do check carefully for complications associated with surgical cannulation (see earlier discussion).

⊗   Do not separate from CPB until ABG, electrolyte, and hematocrit values are satisfactory.

✓   Do have blood products available (coagulopathy is common post-CPB).

CONTROVERSIES

- It is unclear whether IV steroids should be administered in order to attenuate the stress response associated with CPB, and if so, what dose is optimal.
- There is evidence to suggest the superiority of pH-stat rather than alpha-stat management during deep hypothermia, but it is inconclusive.
- Aprotinin is no longer used because of reports of renal failure in adults undergoing cardiac surgery. It is uncertain when and how antifibrinolytics such as aminocaproic acid or tranexamic acid should be used in pediatric cardiac surgery.

SURGICAL CONCERNS

The high flow rate necessary in young pediatric patients often makes surgery technically difficult. Arterial and venous cannulation can also be technically challenging, as discussed earlier, particularly in neonates or in the setting of complex congenital heart disease.

FACTOID

ASD repair was the first successful repair of a cardiac lesion using CPB on May 6, 1953, in Jefferson Medical College Hospital by Dr. John Heysham Gibbon, Jr., who also invented the first CPB machine (known as the "Model II heart-lung device").

14 VENTRICULAR SEPTUM DEFECT REPAIR

Philipp J. Houck, MD

YOUR PATIENT

A 2-month-old patient with a nonrestrictive ventricular septum defect (VSD), pulmonary edema, and congestive heart failure (CHF) presents for VSD closure.

PREOPERATIVE CONSIDERATIONS

There are several kinds of VSDs:

- Perimembranous = paramembranous = membranous = infracristal VSD, most common.
- Subarterial VSD.
- Inlet defects = atrioventricular canal-type VSD.
- Muscular VSDs, often multiple, are in the trabecular portion of the ventricular septum.
- Ventral septal defects can be isolated lesions or part of complex malformations.

Smaller VSDs are restrictive with a pressure gradient across the defect; the shunt is determined by the pressure difference. Larger VSDs are nonrestrictive; the shunt is determined by the relative resistance of the systemic and pulmonary vasculature. Since the pulmonary vascular resistance (PVR) is usually lower than the systemic vascular resistance, pulmonary flow is greater than systemic blood flow and the shunt is left to right.

Infants with nonrestrictive VSDs will increase their shunt as the PVR drops in the first two weeks of life, resulting in pulmonary overcirculation and CHF. Patients frequently have respiratory tract infections and are on diuretics, digitalis, and antibiotics. The overcirculation will then lead to a fixed PVR and end decades later in suprasystemic pulmonary pressures and a shunt reversal (Eisenmenger syndrome) unless the VSD is closed.

Infants with a restrictive VSD may be asymptomatic. Spontaneous closure of VSDs, particularly perimembranous VSDs, can occur.

ANESTHETIC MANAGEMENT

- If the patient has CHF, a primary narcotic technique may be chosen.
- Decrease pulmonary blood flow by avoiding hyperventilation and decreasing fraction of inspired oxygen (FiO_2) for patients with non-restrictive VSDs.
- In patients with pulmonary hypertension, avoid hypercarbia and acidosis.
- Cardiopulmonary bypass with bicaval and aortic cannulation.
- Two IVs, aline, with or without a central line.

POSTOPERATIVE CONSIDERATIONS

Pulmonary hypertension can be seen after the repair of large, isolated ventricular septum defects.

DOs and DON'Ts

✓ Do treat junctional ectopic and supraventricular tachycardia aggressively.

✓ Do treat postoperative pulmonary hypertension with intravenous vasodilators or inhaled nitric oxide.

⊗ Do not needlessly increase the FiO_2 in patients with nonrestrictive VSDs; you may increase the shunt by lowering the PVR.

⊗ Do not overventilate patients with nonrestrictive VSDs; hypocarbia will lower the PVR and increase the shunt.

✓ Do diurese infants prior to extubation and for 1-3 days after the procedure.

✓ Do consider extubation of older and uncomplicated patients.

CONTROVERSIES

Percutaneous closure of a VSD is not as straightforward as ASD closure; it is most commonly done for muscular VSDs.

SURGICAL CONCERNS

Large defects or defects that caused CHF are repaired in infancy; moderate-size VSDs are usually followed up until 5 years of age. Small VSDs are medically managed, but endocarditis prophylaxis is still warranted. Surgical repair is usually through the right atrium and the tricuspid valve, rarely through a right ventriculotomy.

FACTOID

Hippocrates first described ventricular septal defects. Eisenmenger described the shunt reversal in 1897.

15 TETRALOGY OF FALLOT

Anthony J. Clapcich, MD

YOUR PATIENT

A 2-month-old infant diagnosed with tetralogy of Fallot (TOF) at birth is scheduled for repair of large, bilateral inguinal hernias. The parents report only occasional episodes of cyanosis with crying and feeding. The physical exam reveals hypertelorism, bulbous nose, small mouth, cleft palate, and mild retrognathia. Labs: Hematocrit (HCT) 40.

PREOPERATIVE CONSIDERATIONS

TOF is classically defined as follows: (1) right ventricular (RV) outflow tract obstruction (RVOTO) secondary to infundibular narrowing, valvar hypoplasia, and/or pulmonary artery hypoplasia; (2) RV hypertrophy; (3) ventral septum defect (VSD); (4) overriding aorta. Pathophysiology will depend on the degree and direction of shunting that occurs at the VSD level, which in turn is determined by the structural anatomy and by dynamic changes in pulmonary vascular resistance (PVR) and systemic vascular resistance (SVR).

- "Blue tet": stable blood oxygen saturations (SpO_2; high 70s-low 80s), because the presence of severe RVOTO (eg, pulmonary atresia) requires major right-to-left (R-to-L) shunting across the VSD, mixing of oxygenated and deoxygenated blood in the left ventricle, and flow to the pulmonary arteries via a widely patent ductus arteriosus or aortopulmonary collateral.
- "Pink tet": anatomy favors near-normal flow across the RVOT with little R-to-L shunting, more prone to episodes of desaturation or "tet spells" during periods of infundibular spasming or fluctuations in PVR or SVR.

TOF is the most common cardiac lesion seen in children with chromosome 22q11 deletion, which is strongly associated with DiGeorge syndrome, velocardiofacial syndrome, and conotruncal anomaly face syndrome. These patients are at risk for endocrine (hypocalcemia); ear, nose, and throat (cleft palate, feeding and speech difficulties), neurologic (retardation, learning disabilities, motor and speech delays), renal (absent, dysplastic, or multicystic kidneys), hematologic (thrombocytopenia), and autoimmune (T-cell defects, immunodeficiency) abnormalities.

The patient described here appears to have dysmorphic features consistent with chromosome 22q11 deletion. Preoperative studies should include serum calcium, complete blood count, T-cell studies, immunoglobulins, renal ultrasound, electrocardiogram, chest x-ray, and echocardiogram. Feeding issues may be related to a cleft palate or cardiovascular instability. Although the parents report only occasional cyanosis, the relatively elevated HCT (at 2 months, HCT is often 28-30 due to physiologic anemia of infancy) may indicate more frequent episodes of cyanosis with a compensatory increase in hemoglobin production.

ANESTHETIC MANAGEMENT

- Minimize the nothing by mouth period and correct fluid deficits early. The hypertrophied and poorly compliant RV is sensitive to hypovolemia, which can lead to hypotension and increased R-to-L shunting.
- Prepare for possible difficult intubation in patients with facial and/or airway dysmorphism consistent with chromosome 22q11 deletion.
- Avoid agents or techniques that lower SVR and increase R-to-L shunting.
- Avoid hypercarbia, hypoxemia, and acidosis, which can increase PVR and lead to increased R-to-L shunting.
- Avoid hypothermia, as this may increase PVR and lead to increased R-to-L shunting.
- Formulate and initiate an age-appropriate pain control regimen to avoid pain-induced increased PVR and subsequent R-to-L shunting.

Therapeutic maneuvers for "tet spells" include:

- *Knee-chest positioning:* Increases SVR and increases preload by moving blood from peripheral to central compartment.
- *Oxygen:* Decreases PVR, which promotes flow across RVOT and decreases R-to-L shunting across the VSD.
- *Fluid bolus:* Increased preload improves RV mechanics given baseline hypertrophy and decreased compliance.
- *α-1 agonists:* Agents such as phenylephrine and norepinephrine increase SVR and decrease R-to-L shunting.
- *Opioids:* Intramuscular (IM) or intravenous (IV) opioids can decrease circulating catecholamines, decrease PVR, and decrease R-to-L shunting.
- *Ketamine:* IM or IV dissociative anesthetic (decreases anxiety, crying, or screaming) has no effect on PVR in children, but increases SVR and decreases R-to-L shunting.
- *Beta blockers:* Agents such as propranolol can decrease infundibular spasming, improve flow across the RVOT, and thus decrease R-to-L shunting.

POSTOPERATIVE CONSIDERATIONS

- Most patients can be safely monitored in a cardiology unit with experienced nursing staff; patients that exhibit severe and prolonged tet spells should be managed in the intensive care unit.
- Maintain good pain control and normothermia to avoid elevations in PVR.
- Adjust IV fluids and advance feeding by mouth as tolerated to maintain normovolemia and avoid hypotension.

DOs and DON'Ts

✓ Do consider premedication with oral midazolam (even in infants) to decrease crying, screaming, and marked increases in circulating catecholamines.

⊗ Don't cause an iatrogenic air embolus with air bubbles from the IV delivery system during periods of R-to-L shunting.

✓ Do consider adding IM ketamine to the induction regimen to increase SVR and decrease R-to-L shunting.

⊗ Don't use isoflurane for maintenance, as this may decrease SVR and increase R-to-L shunting.

CONTROVERSIES

- *Use of sevoflurane.* Halothane's unique cardiovascular properties (no change in SVR, blunts carotid sinus reflex, strong myocardial depressant that decreases infundibular spasming) made it an ideal anesthetic for TOF. Unfortunately, halothane is now unavailable in the United States, and sevoflurane remains the only widely used agent for mask induction. Sevoflurane can decrease SVR (although to a lesser extent than isoflurane) and promote R-to-L shunting, so the anesthesiologist must be ready to intervene with other modalities if a tet spell is initiated.
- *Neuraxial techniques.* Vasodilation of the venous capacitance vessels with subsequent decrease in preload and arterial vasodilation with subsequent decrease in SVR can accompany blockade of sympathetic fibers arising from T5-L1. Compared to adult patients, infants and young children often demonstrate milder hemodynamic changes secondary to sympathetic nervous system immaturity. However, compared with an adult patient with extensive aortopulmonary collaterals, a pink tet may respond very differently to even mild changes in preload and SVR.

SURGICAL CONCERNS

Physiologic changes associated with laparoscopic herniorrhaphy may precipitate a tet spell. Insufflation of the peritoneum with CO_2 can lead to displacement of the diaphragm, decreased functional residual capacity, decreased lung compliance, increased ventilation/perfusion mismatching, increased atelectasis, increased peak inspiratory pressure, and increased partial pressure of carbon dioxide, which can lead to adverse changes in PVR; increased intra-abdominal pressure can affect inspiratory vital capacity flow, decrease preload, and lead to hypotension with R-to-L shunting in the hypertrophied and poorly compliant RV. An open approach may be a better option.

FACTOID

The harsh systolic murmur that is auscultated along the left upper sternal border is a reflection of the turbulent flow of blood across the narrow RVOT—*not* of flow across the VSD. During a tet spell, there is decreased flow across the RVOTO, increased R-to-L shunting across the VSD, and decreased murmur intensity. Murmur intensity will increase with successful treatment and return of favorable hemodynamics.

16 SINGLE VENTRICLE PHYSIOLOGY

Riva R. Ko, MD

YOUR PATIENT

A 2-year-old boy with a history of hypoplastic left heart syndrome (HLHS), status post Norwood-Sano procedure and bidirectional Glenn shunt (BDG), presents for Fontan operation. History is otherwise unremarkable.

> *Meds*: Digoxin, aspirin
> *Labs*: Hemoglobin (Hgb) 17.1
> *Physical exam*: Clubbing, cyanosis. $SpO_2 = 80\%$

PREOPERATIVE CONSIDERATIONS

Patients with single ventricle physiology, usually due to HLHS or tricuspid atresia, require staged surgical palliation, ultimately resulting in passive delivery of deoxygenated blood to the pulmonary circulation (bypassing the ventricle) and delivery of oxygenated blood to the systemic circulation via the single ventricle. In the neonatal period, a patent ductus arteriosus (PDA) provides systemic blood flow in patients with HLHS, so prostaglandin E1 is used in order to maintain the PDA patent and improve the pulmonary and systemic blood flows (Qp/Qs) until surgical palliation can be performed. The usual first-stage palliation for neonates with HLHS is the Norwood procedure, which entails the creation of a neo-aorta from the hypoplastic aorta and the main pulmonary artery (PA), thereby connecting the right ventricle (RV) to the systemic circulation. Pulmonary blood flow is maintained by the creation of either a modified Blalock-Taussig shunt (a Gore-Tex patch from the neo-aorta to the RPA) or, as in this case, a Sano modification (a Gore-Tex patch from the RV to the PA). The second-stage palliation for HLHS patients, the BDG, establishes blood flow from the SVC to the right and left PAs; this is done in order to decrease the exposure of the pulmonary circulation to the volume overload of a systemic arterial-to-PA shunt. The BDG is usually performed at around 6 months of age, when PVR has decreased, but it can be done as early as 2-3 months. The Fontan operation is the third and final stage of palliation for patients with HLHS, and generally is undertaken at between 2 and 4 years of age. In the Fontan procedure, the inferior vena cava (IVC) is connected to the PA, establishing a total cavopulmonary connection. The IVC-PA anastomosis can be accomplished either via an intra-atrial lateral tunnel or via an extracardiac conduit to the PA. A fenestration between the single atrium and the Fontan connections is frequently performed in order to decrease venous pressure and to allow for adequate ventricular volume loading.

Patients normally will have a transthoracic echocardiogram as well as a cardiac catheterization preoperatively to determine their readiness for completion of the Fontan operation. In addition to evaluation of the patient's functional clinical status, preoperative evaluation should include a thorough assessment of these data, with emphasis on adequacy of valvular function, ventricular end-diastolic pressures, and transpulmonary pressure gradient. A careful neuro-logic history should be taken, as there is risk of systemic stroke due to venous emboli in patients who have undergone BDG. Parents should be informed that there is significant risk of venous throm-bosis and central nervous system complications after the Fontan operation.

Patients presenting for the Fontan operation have already been through at least two major surgeries as well as cardiac catheterizations under general anesthesia, so premedication with oral midazolam can be helpful in alleviating anxiety.

ANESTHETIC MANAGEMENT

- Inhalation or IV induction of anesthesia is acceptable. Unlike in the adult population, nitrous oxide and ketamine do not cause elevation of PVR in children and can be used safely.
- Give high doses of narcotic prior to laryngoscopy to prevent increases in PVR.
- Place arterial line after induction, usually radial if possible.
- Obtain good IV access. Placement of a central venous line is contro-versial (see Controversies in this chapter). Make sure blood is available prior to incision.
- Maintain anesthesia with IV narcotics and muscle relaxants, with or without low concentrations of inhalational agents.
- Consider intraoperative loading and infusion of aminocaproic acid to decrease bleeding.
- Use intraoperative transesophageal echocardiography (TEE) to assess volume status, ventricular contractility, atrioventricular (AV) valvular function, and patency of anastomoses.

- Post-CPB, maintain central venous pressure (CVP) at about 14-20 mm Hg in order to preserve adequate pulmonary perfusion and cardiac output. Replace surgical blood loss with cell saver and/or blood as necessary.
- Administer blood products as needed to promote coagulation (platelets, cryoprecipitate, fresh frozen plasma).
- Because of the absence of RV contractility and passive pulmonary blood flow, it is imperative to prevent increases in either PVR or SVR. Maintain high fraction of inspired oxygen (FiO_2) in combination with hyperventilation to decrease PVR. Ventilator settings should include a shortened inspiratory time and prolonged expiratory time. Although low inspiratory pressures are indicated, consider low-dose positive end-expiratory pressure in patients with atelectasis. Strongly consider using inhaled nitric oxide (iNO) in patients having difficulty weaning from CPB.
- Plan for hemodynamic support post-CPB, usually with an inotropic agent such as milrinone, as well as pressure support with an agent such as epinephrine. The goal is to increase inotropy and decrease SVR and PVR, thereby minimizing impedance to ejection and optimizing preload. Patients frequently require diuresis.
- Keep patients in sinus rhythm in order to preserve ventricular preload and cardiac output. This may require placement of pacing wires by the surgeon.
- Timing of extubation must weigh the benefits of improved systemic venous return associated with spontaneous ventilation against the risks of persistent hypoxia, hypercarbia, and atelectasis with resultant increased PVR.

POSTOPERATIVE CONSIDERATIONS

Patients generally are transported intubated to the intensive care unit, with consideration being given to early extubation when feasible (see previous discussion). Some degree of hypoxemia is to be expected, particularly in patients with a fenestrated Fontan; however, systemic oxygen desaturation <85% may indicate excessive flow across the fenestration or the existence of pulmonary arteriovenous malformations. Inadequate volume must be replaced immediately, either with blood or with crystalloids. Electrolytes must be checked and corrected as necessary to prevent myocardial dysfunction. Pacing should be instituted in patients with arrhythmias. Inotropic, pressor, and iNO support are weaned as tolerated. Pleural and pericardial effusions are common in the postoperative period, and usually can be treated with drainage, diuresis, and volume replacement. Prolonged effusions may necessitate cardiac catheterization to rule out a treatable cause, such as baffle obstruction or innominate vein thrombosis.

DOs and DON'Ts

✓   Do premedicate anxious patients with oral midazolam.
✓   Do use generous doses of IV narcotics for intubation and maintenance of anesthesia.
✓   Do make sure to secure adequate IV access. Placement of a central venous line is controversial.
✓   Do use intraoperative TEE to assess volume status, function, and adequacy of repair.
⊗   Do not allow patients to become hypovolemic. Maintain CVP at about 14-20 mm Hg. Transfuse as needed.
⊗   Do not allow PVR to increase; use high FiO_2, hyperventilation, and low inspiratory pressures. Use iNO as necessary.
⊗   Do not allow patients to remain in a nonsinus rhythm. Use pacing as needed.
✓   Do implement hemodynamic support, particularly inotropy, post-CPB.
✓   Do consider early extubation when possible to minimize the negative effects of positive pressure ventilation (decreased systemic venous return, increased PVR).

CONTROVERSIES

- Although CVP monitoring is helpful for patients undergoing the Fontan procedure, the site of catheter placement is controversial. Both the internal jugular (IJ) and the femoral veins have the potential for thrombosis; moreover, right IJ placement may interfere with the Glenn anastomosis, while femoral veins may be scarred from prior cardiac catheterizations. The decision as to whether or not to place a central venous line in Fontan patients, and if so, where, must be made on an individual basis; this decision also may be affected by the adequacy of peripheral IV access. In the absence of a central line, the surgeon will often place one or more right atrial lines for administration of pressors and measurement of central pressures.
- It is controversial whether or not to discontinue digoxin one day prior to surgery in light of the potential derangements in serum potassium associated with CPB and the potential for ventricular arrhythmias.

SURGICAL CONCERNS

As mentioned previously, the surgeon frequently places a fenestration to allow for improved cardiac output, albeit at the expense of mildly decreased systemic saturation. Temporary pacing wires normally are placed because of the high incidence of postoperative dysrhythmias. Theoretically, an extracardiac Fontan may result in a lower incidence of dysrhythmias than a lateral tunnel due to fewer suture lines and avoidance of RA hypertension. In the event of systemic venous desaturation post-CPB, a baffle leak or an excessively large fenestration must be considered. Low cardiac output post-CPB, particularly in the setting of elevated LA pressure, may be indicative of AV valve regurgitation or of ventricular dysfunction and/or outflow obstruction, which may require surgical repair.

FACTOID

Originally, the Fontan operation was proposed in the early 1970s as an operative treatment for tricuspid atresia; it was later expanded to include other single ventricle lesions. Initial attempts at one-stage complete Fontan circulation resulted in universal mortality as a result of insufficient RV function and/or compromised coronary blood flow. This led to the principle of staged reconstruction for patients with single-ventricle lesions, which was developed and refined by William Norwood.

17 PULMONARY HYPERTENSION

Arthur J. Smerling, MD

YOUR PATIENT

A 12-year-old girl presents with dyspnea on exertion, chest pain, syncope, and a murmur. She is scheduled for a diagnostic cardiac catheterization.

> *Physical exam*: Thin girl, loud P2, right-sided gallop, pulsatile liver.
> *Chest x-ray*: Large central pulmonary arteries (PAs), oligemic lung fields.
> *Echocardiogram*: Tricuspid regurgitation, significant TR jet, right ventricular (RV) hypertrophy, and a septum that bulges into the left ventricle during systole.

PREOPERATIVE CONSIDERATIONS

Pulmonary hypertension (PH) is defined as mean pulmonary arterial pressure >25 mm Hg at rest and may be associated with familial, endocrine, cardiac, hepatic, thrombotic, HIV, pulmonary, or rheumatologic disease. The onset of symptoms is often insidious; the dyspnea is often misdiagnosed as asthma, and the syncope is confused with seizures. The incidence is higher in populations living at high altitude, and it occurs more often in females than in males. Physiologically, PH patients with left-to-right shunts have too much blood flow, while PH patients with increased pre- or postcapillary resistance have too little blood flow. Increased precapillary resistance may be associated with vascular obstruction, constriction, or obliteration. Inhaled nitric oxide (iNO) is beneficial only in precapillary constriction. iNO will increase the flow in left-to-right shunts and cause pulmonary edema in patients with postcapillary resistance.

ANESTHETIC MANAGEMENT

- Benzodiazepine premedication is recommended to blunt catecholamine surge.
- Upper respiratory tract infection will increase risk and also make the data unreliable—postpone the case.
- Narcotics, benzodiazepines, IV sedatives, and potent agents are acceptable, but avoid hypoventilation and hypotension.

- Avoid increases in intrathoracic pressure, eg, through coughing, straining, or Valsalva maneuver.
- Even a small degree of hypoxia, hypercarbia, acidosis, catecholamine release, or airway obstruction will raise PA pressure. Monitor O_2 saturation and end-tidal CO_2 closely.
- Once the sheath is placed, you can decrease the amount of anesthetic.
- Maintain coronary perfusion. If you cannot lower the RV pressure, raise the mean arterial pressure.
- If the patient is on a continuous prostaglandin infusion, do not interrupt it.
- Patients with atrial communications will shunt right to left and desaturate but will not arrest during a pulmonary hypertensive crisis.
- In case of hypotension, consider administering vasopressin as a systemic vasoconstrictor.
- Death during the procedure is often due to RV ischemia or pulmonary hemorrhage. Monitor the electrocardiogram for signs of ischemia (especially bradycardia) and the fluoroscopy for signs of hemorrhage.

POSTOPERATIVE CONSIDERATIONS

- Continue to avoid the Valsalva maneuver.
- If the patient develops a pulmonary hemorrhage, sedate, paralyze, and consider one lung ventilation.

DOs and DON'Ts

⊗   Avoid platelet transfusions. The serotonin increases PA pressure.

⊗   Avoid coughing during the extubation; consider deep extubation if the patient has a good airway.

✓   Oxygen will often lower PA pressure in patients with congestive heart disease or chronic lung disease.

✓   iNO will often lower PA pressure in patients with idiopathic PH.

CONTROVERSIES

- Spontaneous ventilation allows the most relevant evaluation, but it may be difficult to avoid airway obstruction, hypercarbia, and catecholamine surges.
- A nasal cannula can be used to monitor CO_2 and to administer oxygen and iNO. If the patient needs airway support, a laryngeal mask airway is usually tolerated better than an endotracheal tube. If the patient

deteriorates, intubate and consider pulmonary hemorrhage or RV failure.
- Many practitioners avoid ketamine because it may increase PA pressures.

SURGICAL CONCERNS

- Inflating the PA balloon may decrease pulmonary blood flow, decrease saturation, and increase RV afterload—be vigilant!

FACTOIDS

- The most common cause of pulmonary hypertension in developing countries is schistosomiasis.
- Ortner's syndrome is hoarseness caused by impingement of the left recurrent laryngeal nerve by pressure from the dilated pulmonary artery and other structures.
- Clubbing is associated with PH secondary to cardiac, hepatic, or pulmonary parenchymal disease that is not familial or idiopathic.

18 CARDIAC CATHETERIZATION AFTER HEART TRANSPLANTATION

Philipp J. Houck, MD

YOUR PATIENT

A 7-year-old girl presents for her annual heart catheterization with endomyocardial biopsies. She was transplanted 3 years ago for dilated cardiomyopathy.

PREOPERATIVE CONSIDERATIONS

After the first year posttransplant, when there are multiple biopsies, most patients undergo biopsies every 6 months and get annual coronary angiography.

Preoperative evaluation should include review of the electrocardiogram, echocardiogram, and available data from prior catheterizations. Cardiac function, recent labs, and the presence of allograft vasculopathy should be known. Ischemia can be silent because of the surgical denervation.

Right ventricular failure is seen in the immediate postoperative period for patients who had elevated pulmonary pressures before the transplant. The pretransplant cardiac history typically becomes less relevant as time progresses.

Kidney failure and hypertension are frequently seen in this population.

The psychological aspect of having repeated procedures and a life-threatening disease cannot be underestimated. Respecting specific requests for the anesthesiologists gives patients and their families a sense of autonomy and enhances the satisfaction of both.

ANESTHETIC MANAGEMENT

- Most anesthesiologists and patients prefer mask inductions because in this patient group, obtaining intravenous access can be very challenging. If no access is obtainable, one has the option of relying on the access that the cardiologist establishes for the procedure.
- Sedation is possible with compliant and motivated patients. Normocarbia is desired for hemodynamic measurements, and this often makes general anesthesia with a laryngeal mask airway or an endotracheal tube necessary.

- The denervated heart relies on an intact Frank-Starling mechanism and circulating catecholamines.
- Maintenance of anesthesia on room air is preferable to mimic the usual hemodynamic state.
- Deep extubation is preferred to avoid bleeding from arterial or venous puncture sites from movement during extubation.
- The transplanted heart is denervated and will not respond to indirectly acting catecholamines.

POSTOPERATIVE CONSIDERATIONS

Patients need to keep their leg with the arterial cannulation site straight for up to 6 hours. This is difficult to achieve in smaller children without sedation.

DOs and DON'Ts

✓   Do treat hypotension with fluid boluses.
⊗   Do not start IVs on extremities that are being cannulated, unless you have to.
✓   Do inform the cardiologist if you are giving vasoactive medications, since this will change the hemodynamic measurements.
⊗   Do not give large amounts of neostigmine—the patient may develop bradycardia or arrest.
⊗   Do not give a stress dose of steroids, unless clinically needed.
✓   Be prepared for cardiac arrest at any time, particularly when the coronaries are manipulated. Manipulation of the coronaries in children can easily lead to vasospasm and ischemia.

SURGICAL CONCERNS

About 50% of all retransplantations are for posttransplant coronary vasculopathies. Endomyocardial biopsies are done to screen for rejection. Hemodynamic measurements are changed by acute pulmonary illness, another argument for not undergoing these often elective procedures in patients with active upper respiratory tract infections.

FACTOID

Gene expression profiling of peripheral blood samples could replace endomyocardial biopsies in the future.

PART 3

RESPIRATORY

19 ASTHMA

Gracie M. Almeida-Chen, MD, MPH

YOUR PATIENT

A 15-year-old male with asthma develops intraoperative bronchospasm.

PREOPERATIVE CONSIDERATIONS

The goal of preoperative assessment in an asthmatic patient is to gauge the severity and control of the asthma. Key factors in determining the severity of the asthma are:

- Number of acute exacerbations, hospital presentations, and admissions in a year
- Recent asthma symptoms, medical interventions, and hospital visits
- Level of maintenance therapy
- Albuterol frequency, recent use, and recent escalation of therapy
- Number of episodes of oral corticosteroid use for acute exacerbations within the past year
- Previous intensive care admission and invasive ventilation
- Any specific triggers for bronchospasm
- Presence of recent cold symptoms within the last two weeks
- Functional exercise tolerance is a useful marker of severity

A patient with severe asthmatic attacks is more likely to develop perioperative bronchospasm and would benefit from a preoperative consultation with a pulmonologist to optimize his or her asthma control.

Common triggers for childhood asthma exacerbation include the following:

- Upper respiratory infection (URI)—usually viral
- Smoke or other inhaled irritant gases
- Pollen
- Foreign bodies

Potential trigger agents should be identified and avoided. The usual inhaled and oral medications should be taken the day of surgery.

ANESTHETIC MANAGEMENT

- A patient with a history of prolonged oral prednisolone or high dose of inhaled corticosteroids within the previous 12 months may benefit from a single intraoperative dose of corticosteroids.
- Consider a premedication to avoid or reduce the patient's anxiety upon induction. Crying or coughing during uncooperative inhalational induction may trigger acute bronchospasm.
- A deep plane of anesthesia reduces airway reactivity associated with intubation.
- Avoid carinal irritation, which may precipitate bronchospasm.
- Avoid irritant volatile agents (desflurane), which may precipitate bronchospasm.
- Consider the total intravenous anesthesia (TIVA) technique and regional anesthesia.
- Consider using ketamine for IV induction (1-2 mg/kg) and maintenance (12.5-45 µg/kg/min infusion) of anesthesia.

Intraoperative management of bronchospasm

- Ensure adequate oxygen delivery and carbon dioxide clearance.
- Eliminate mechanical causes: blocked or kinked endotracheal tube (ETT), carinal irritation, or a defective circuit.
- Eliminate other causes of increased airway pressures: pneumothorax, abdominal splinting due to light anesthesia, or anaphylaxis.
- Limit ventilator pressures to reduce risk of barotraumas and cardiovascular collapse: increase fraction of inspired oxygen (FiO_2), reduce respiratory rate, reduce inspiratory:expiratory (I:E) ratio (prolong expiratory time to avoid gas trapping).
- Deepen the level of anesthesia with volatile agents or with propofol.
- Inhaled albuterol (metered-dose inhaler [MDI] + spacer): up to 10 puffs (1 mg) every 20-30 minutes.
- Subcutaneous terbutaline 10 µg/kg (maximum dose of 250 µg).
- Aminophylline: 5-7 mg/kg IV over 30 minutes followed by a 0.5-1.5 mg/kg/h infusion.
- Corticosteroids:
  - Hydrocortisone 4 mg/kg IV
  - Methylprednisone 1 mg/kg IV
- Epinephrine (1:1000) IV: 1-10 mcg/kg:
  - Subcutaneous: 10 µg/kg (maximum dose of 400 µg)
  - ETT: 1 µg/kg
- Magnesium: 40 mg/kg IV over 20 minutes.
- Volatile anesthetic agents.

POSTOPERATIVE CONSIDERATIONS

- Deep extubation
- Postoperative intensive care unit monitoring

DOs and DON'Ts

✓ Do optimize the patient prior to surgery.
✓ Do wait for the patient to have a deep level of anesthesia prior to instrumenting the airway.
⊗ Do not irritate the carina.

CONTROVERSIES

ETT versus laryngeal mask airway (LMA). Data show that supraglottic devices are preferred in patients with upper respiratory tract infections. Tracheal intubation is believed to be more likely to produce adverse respiratory events in an asthmatic patient than the use of an LMA. This has not been investigated directly in children. However, LMA insertion may also produce bronchospasm, especially in a patient who has not reached an adequate depth of anesthesia, and it is more difficult to manage the consequent ventilatory requirements without an ETT.

SURGICAL CONCERNS

Surgery should be delayed in a patient with poor asthma control, recent or current URI, or lower respiratory tract infection. Airway hyperreactivity related to a viral URI persists for approximately 4 weeks.

FACTOID

Worldwide, asthma is estimated to occur in 300 million people and is implicated in 1 of every 250 deaths. Its prevalence in the United States is 6.7% of the population and 12% of children. It is the leading cause of chronic illness in children.

Chronic wheezing can sometimes also be related to an aspirated foreign body.

20 BRONCHOPULMONARY DYSPLASIA

Gracie M. Almeida-Chen, MD, MPH

YOUR PATIENT

A 4-month-old, former 28-week premie with bronchopulmonary dysplasia (BPD) presents for eye surgery.

PREOPERATIVE CONSIDERATIONS

Bronchopulmonary dysplasia, the most common cause of chronic lung disease in infants, is a disease of small airways and lung parenchyma, characterized by abnormal growth of alveoli and vasculature, and dilation of distal sites of gas exchange (alveolar ducts). It is the consequence of both oxygen toxicity and ventilator-induced lung injury to immature lungs.

Bronchopulmonary dysplasia is a clinical diagnosis based on oxygen requirement and the need for ventilator support. It results when neonates with respiratory distress syndrome develop persistent respiratory distress characterized by airway obstruction, increased airway reactivity and resistance, and lung hyperinflation. This results in a ventilation-to-perfusion mismatch, reduced pulmonary compliance, increased work of breathing, and compromised gas exchange, leading to hypoxia, hypercarbia, tachypnea, and, in severe cases, right heart failure, resulting in pulmonary hypertension and ultimately cor pulmonale. The clinical manifestations are rapid respiration, wheezing, cough, and frequent episodes of fever, desaturation, and bradycardia. Oxygen consumption is increased by as much as 25%. Failure to thrive is a sign of chronic hypoxia. Auscultation of the lungs may not reveal wheezing because the site of airway hyperactivity is primarily in the small airways at the periphery of the lungs as a result of increased thickness of the airway wall.

Infants with mild forms of BPD improve with age and may become asymptomatic, but airway hyperreactivity may persist. Most infants with moderate to severe BPD remain oxygen dependent, with or without ventilator dependence, beyond 4 weeks of age. Maintenance of adequate oxygenation, with partial pressure of oxygen (PaO_2) >55 mm Hg and oxygen saturation (SpO_2) >94%, is necessary to prevent or treat cor pulmonale and to promote growth of lung tissue and remodeling of the pulmonary vascular bed. Reactive airway bronchoconstriction is treated with bronchodilating agents and steroids. Cor pulmonale and severe chest retractions that draw fluid into the interstitial space cause fluid retention, necessitating fluid restriction and diuretic administration in order to decrease pulmonary edema and improve gas exchange. Consequently, abnormal serum electrolyte levels (eg, hypokalemia, hypochloremia, or metabolic alkalosis) are common preoperatively.

ANESTHETIC MANAGEMENT

- Obtain a baseline oxygen saturation measurement with a pulse oximeter prior to administering an anesthetic. A normal oxygen saturation level does not guarantee the absence of lung dysfunction.
- Arterial saturation should be maximized to reduce pulmonary hypertension.
- Desaturation may be rapid when apnea occurs.
- Infants with BPD with near-normal SpO_2 on room air may develop marked desaturation after induction with sevoflurane because of a loss of hypoxic pulmonary vasoconstriction under general anesthesia.
- Avoid nitrous oxide to avoid exacerbation of pulmonary gas trapping and pulmonary vascular resistance.
- In children with a history of mechanical ventilation, an endotracheal tube (ETT) one size smaller than the appropriate-sized ETT for the patient's age should be available, as subglottic stenosis may be present.
- Subglottic stenosis, tracheomalacia, and bronchomalacia may also be present as sequelae of prolonged intubation.
- The possible presence of airway hyperactivity and increased risk of bronchospasm warrants establishing a surgical level of anesthesia before instrumenting the airway. Instrumentation of the airway may also be associated with pulmonary, as well as systemic, hypertension.
- These children may also have reactive airway disease and should be treated similarly to those with asthma. Perioperative bronchodilator therapy should be considered.
- Patients may require increased respiratory support intraoperatively, including increased peak airway pressures, positive end-expiratory pressure, and oxygen concentrations, to maintain baseline oxygenation and ventilation. However, high airway pressures may cause pneumothorax.
- Adequate oxygen should be delivered to maintain a PaO_2 of 50-70 mm Hg.
- Patients with metabolic alkalosis from furosemide therapy may exhibit a compensatory retention of CO_2.
- Hyperventilation of patients with compensated metabolic alkalosis may cause hypotension from severe alkalosis.
- Fluid administration should be monitored and minimized to avoid pulmonary edema.

POSTOPERATIVE CONSIDERATIONS

- Infants with BPD are at increased risk of developing coughing, laryngospasm, bronchospasm, atelectasis, pneumonia, and hypoxic episodes during the postoperative period.
- Postoperative mechanical ventilation may be required.

DOs and DON'Ts

✓ Do analyze the infant's current and recent ventilator history, including severity and treatment of airway reactivity.
✓ Do allow for adequate expiratory times, especially in patients with obstructive lung disease.
✓ Do assess the infant's acid-base status (PaCO$_2$, pH, and base deficit) and preoperative hepatic and renal function to determine what kind of and how much fluid to administer during surgery.
⊗ Do not use high peak airway pressures because of the increased risk of pneumothorax, pneumomediastinum, or interstitial emphysema. But you may be surprised by how much pressure is needed to ventilate immediately after the intubation. This can be mistakenly interpreted as an esophageal intubation.
✓ Do reserve an intensive care unit bed for postoperative care in patients with severe BPD.

CONTROVERSIES

There are questions concerning how much of an increase in respiratory support is needed, including higher peak airway pressures, to maintain baseline oxygenation and ventilation. However, high airway pressures may cause pneumothorax.

SURGICAL CONCERNS

The higher peak airway pressures that may be needed to maintain baseline oxygenation and ventilation may cause a pneumothorax.

FACTOID

FACTORS THAT CONTRIBUTE TO THE PATHOGENESIS OF BPD

Factors Associated with Prematurity

- Positive pressure ventilation
- High inspired oxygen concentration

- Inflammation, alone or associated with infection
- Pulmonary edema due to patent ductus arteriosus or excess fluid administration
- Pulmonary air leak
- Nutritional deficiencies
- Airway hyperreactivity
- Early adrenal insufficiency

Other Factors

- Meconium aspiration pneumonia
- Neonatal pneumonia
- Congestive heart disease
- Wilson-Mikity syndrome

21 CROUP

Gracie M. Almeida-Chen, MD, MPH

YOUR PATIENT

A 21-month-old male presents to the emergency room with a several-day history of upper respiratory symptoms, progressing to hoarseness, inspiratory stridor, a "barking" cough, rhinorrhea, and a low-grade fever.

PREOPERATIVE CONSIDERATIONS

LARYNGOTRACHEOBRONCHITIS (SUBGLOTTIC CROUP)

Croup, which affects primarily children between the ages of 6 months and 3 years, is a viral-mediated inflammation that affects the subglottic tracheal mucosa and the tracheobronchial tree. The patient presents with symptoms of upper respiratory infection, including rhinorrhea, cough, sore throat, and low-grade fever for several days before developing symptoms of upper airway obstruction characterized by inspiratory stridor and a barky or seal-like cough. The symptoms may last from a few days to more than a week with varying degrees of severity, and may be worse at night in the supine position.

Croup's etiologies are parainfluenza virus type 1 (the most common), parainfluenza virus types 2 and 3, influenza A and B, respiratory syncytial virus, *Mycoplasma* pneumonia, herpes simplex I, and adenovirus. Although it is a viral illness, some patients may acquire bacterial superinfection of their airway and require antibiotic therapy.

Management of croup consists of humidified air, either heated or cool mist. If symptoms are more severe, nebulized racemic epinephrine can reduce airway edema. Steroid administration is controversial, but may decrease the severity of the disease, decrease the need for tracheal intubation, or hasten improvement in the first 24 hours of illness.

Heliox may be used if other therapies do not provide adequate management. In severe cases of hypoxemia that do not respond to nebulized epinephrine and oxygen therapy, endotracheal intubation is required.

BACTERIAL TRACHEITIS (MEMBRANOUS CROUP)

Bacterial tracheitis (membranous croup) is a rare, potentially life-threatening disease affecting children in a wider range of ages, with the average being 5 years of age. Children present with a more toxic appearance than those with viral laryngotracheobronchitis. They present with stridor, a barking cough, and a temperature greater than 38.5°. An endoscopic exam reveals an inflamed and edematous tracheal wall with thick, tenacious, adherent secretions.

Management consists of initiation of broad-spectrum antibiotic therapy. This should change when cultures and sensitivities are known. An endotracheal tube (ETT) should be placed for frequent tracheal suctioning, with secretions decreasing in 3-5 days. The patient should be initially observed in the intensive care unit even if not intubated.

POSTINTUBATION CROUP

The major cause of postintubation croup is subglottic injury and edema associated with traumatic intubation, especially with an oversized ETT. The incidence of postintubation croup increases when there is no air leak around the ETT and the airway pressure exceeds 40 cm H_2O. Other factors associated with postintubation croup may include traumatic or repeated intubation, "bucking" or coughing with the ETT in place, changing the head position, the duration of surgery, and neck surgery. The incidence of postintubation croup has decreased with the use of an ETT that produces an air leak around the tube with a pressure lower than 30 cm H_2O and with corticosteroids.

Cool, humidified mist administered after extubation may be helpful in mild cases of croup. Racemic epinephrine (0.5 mL of 2.25% solution), diluted in 3-5 mL of normal saline solution and administered by nebulizer for 5-10 minutes, assists patients with progressively worsening symptoms and stridor by producing mucosal vasoconstriction, resulting in a shrinking of swollen airway mucosa. The "rebound effect" and recurrence of symptoms necessitate observing the patient for up to 4 hours after treatment. Dexamethasone is effective in reducing the incidence of postintubation croup in children who have been intubated for longer than 48 hours.

ANESTHETIC MANAGEMENT

- Induction with IV access already obtained is common.
- If no IV is present, use a sevoflurane induction while maintaining spontaneous respirations.
- Routine direct laryngoscopy is performed.

- Symptomatic patients who require intubation of the trachea need an ETT 0.5-1.0 mm smaller in diameter than would be used in children without croup.

POSTOPERATIVE CONSIDERATIONS

- The patient typically remains sedated with an ETT in place for at least 48-96 hours.
- When a leak is present at 20-25 cm H_2O, extubation may be considered.

DOs and DON'Ts

✓ Do observe patients for up to 4 hours after treatment with racemic epinephrine nebulizer because of the "rebound effect" and recurrence of symptoms.
✓ Do intubate with a smaller ETT.

SURGICAL CONCERNS

Tracheotomy is rarely needed as therapy for these patients and is reserved only for unusual cases.

FACTOID

The croup scoring system by Downs and Raphaely objectively quantifies the severity of the condition, and its use can be helpful in treatment decisions (Table 21-1).

A lateral neck radiograph typically shows a narrowing of the airway shadow below the vocal cords. An anteroposterior radiograph of the neck may show a long area of airway narrowing resembling the steeple of a church ("steeple sign").

TABLE 21-1   CLINICAL CROUP SCORE

	Score		
Criteria	0	1	2
Inspiratory breathing sounds	Normal	Harsh with rhonchi	Delayed
Stridor	None	Inspiratory	Inspiratory and expiratory
Cough	None	Hoarse cry	Bark
Retraction and flaring	None	Suprasternal, (+) flaring	Suprasternal, subcostal, intercostal, (+) flaring
Cyanosis (sat <90%)	None	In room air	In 40% oxygen

22 ASPIRATION PNEUMONIA

Manon Haché, MD

YOUR PATIENT

A 14-year-old male patient with developmental delay presents for a Nissen fundoplication and gastrostomy tube. He takes esomeprazole and ranitidine. He has a history of having been born at 27 weeks' gestation, with cerebral palsy, developmental delay, seizure disorder treated by levetiracetam, chronic lung disease, and severe gastroesophageal reflux disease (GERD) with multiple episodes of aspiration pneumonias. He takes fluticasone and albuterol daily. He also takes glycopyrrolate to help with management of copious oral secretions. During your rapid-sequence induction, a large volume of clear liquid is noted in the oropharynx, which you suction before passing your endotracheal tube.

PREOPERATIVE CONSIDERATIONS

Patients with chronic GERD and a history of aspiration pneumonia will come to you with chronic lung disease secondary to multiple episodes of aspiration. Even if they have no documented episodes of aspiration pneumonia, they may have microaspiration and will not have a great pulmonary reserve. We consider them at risk for aspiration during the induction of anesthesia, and should plan to do a rapid-sequence induction (or alternatively, an awake fiberoptic intubation). Patients with severe developmental delay and cerebral palsy will have varying degrees of cognitive dysfunction, and we should be careful when approaching these patients to be sensitive to the fact that they may have a perfect understanding of what is happening around them but be unable to communicate effectively.

ANESTHETIC MANAGEMENT

• Rapid-sequence induction should be favored. Premedication with benzodiazepines is controversial; sometimes, it seems that they are necessary to preoxygenate a patient adequately, and giving patients a small dose of midazolam should not be detrimental to the patient's ability to protect the airway. The risks and benefits of doing this should be weighed.

- Always have suction available when you induce, as a rapid-sequence induction does not guarantee the absence of regurgitation.
- Be ready to treat aspiration with suction and bronchoalveolar lavage if it is noted; bronchoscopy is indicated in the case of particulate aspiration.
- The cricoid maneuver is classic, but the evidence to support its effectiveness is lacking. It may make visualization of the vocal cords harder.
- Succinylcholine is not necessarily contraindicated in patients with cerebral palsy. Their cerebral injury is remote and stable. However, some of them are quite immobile, depending on the severity of their spasticity.

POSTOPERATIVE CONSIDERATIONS

The decision on whether or not to extubate a patient who has suffered aspiration depends on how the patient is doing during the case. If the patient has significant desaturation and is difficult to ventilate, the case should be rescheduled and the patient should be taken to the pediatric intensive care unit for further management of aspiration pneumonia or pneumonitis. More commonly, patients will be asymptomatic, and following bronchoalveolar lavage, the patient will be stable for surgery to continue. If the patient remains stable from a respiratory standpoint, then extubation should be attempted, but the patient should definitely be admitted and watched, as complications may appear later. Patients may develop pneumonitis when the acidic contents aspirated are irritating for the lungs, or pneumonia if the aspiration of the contents was colonized; this is most likely the case if patients present with community acquired pneumonia. Most complicated intraoperative aspiration events will lead to pneumonitis, and antibiotics are not indicated.

DOs and DON'Ts

✓   Do conduct a rapid-sequence induction.
✓   Do treat aspiration with bronchoalveolar lavage and bronchodilators as needed.
⊗   Do not do a mask induction.
✓   Do admit patients postoperatively.
✓   Do cancel the case and stabilize patients who have severe clinical manifestations following aspiration.

CONTROVERSIES

Opioids are not classically part of a rapid-sequence induction, but patients may be more hemodynamically stable when they are used. Some argue that they may remove respiratory drive in the event of a difficult intubation.

Succinylcholine is still the gold standard muscle relaxant to be used for rapid-sequence intubation, but rocuronium at 3 ED95 provides comparable intubating conditions when a contraindication is present.

SURGICAL CONCERNS

It used to be that a patient getting a gastrostomy tube would almost automatically get a Nissen fundoplication to decrease the risk of reflux. Now, this decision is made on a case-by-case basis depending on the indication for the gastrostomy tube. Some patients have oral and/or pharyngeal dysfunction that causes feeding difficulties and are not necessarily at risk for regurgitation, and thus they may never need a Nissen fundoplication.

FACTOID

Historically, it was thought that the volume of aspiration was important when assessing the severity of symptoms that would occur after aspiration, with 0.4 mL/kg of acidic volume being quoted as putting the patient at risk for pneumonitis. We learned later that this volume had been directly injected into the right mainstem bronchus of only one monkey, causing pneumonitis. It is in fact not known how much or what pH puts a patient at risk for pneumonitis, as alkaline products are also very irritating to the lungs.

23 PULMONARY SEQUESTRATION

Leila M. Pang, MD
Manon Haché, MD

YOUR PATIENT

An otherwise healthy 8-year-old male with a history of repeated pulmonary infections is scheduled for a thoracoscopic resection of a sequestered lung.

PREOPERATIVE CONSIDERATIONS

Sequestration of the lung can occur as a cystic or solid mass composed of nonfunctioning pulmonary tissue that does not connect to the tracheo-bronchial tree. Symptomatic patients usually present with recurrent pulmonary infections, while asymptomatic patients may be diagnosed from a routine chest radiograph. Two forms of sequestered lungs can be found. Intrapulmonary sequestration is a segment surrounded by normal lung tissue, with its blood supply from systemic vessels and drainage into the pulmonary veins. Extrapulmonary sequestration will have only its pleural sac, with the vascular supply being exclusively from the systemic system.

Other anomalies are rare (<10%) with intrapulmonary sequestration, while foregut communication and other anomalies such as congenital diaphragmatic hernia, congenital adenomatoid malformations, and congenital heart disease are more common with extrapulmonary sequestration (about 50% of the cases). Extrapulmonary sequestration is more commonly diagnosed in infancy during the workup of the other congenital anomalies.

Other congenital lung lesions that may require surgical interventions are congenital cystic adenomatoid malformation and congenital lobar emphysema.

ANESTHETIC MANAGEMENT

- Use standard American Society of Anesthesiologists monitors and arterial line.
- Ensure adequate IV access.
- Anesthesia induction can be inhalational or intravenous.
- Many surgeons request one-lung ventilation, which may be achieved using either a double-lumen tube (size permitting), a bronchial

blocker, or endobronchial intubation with a regular endotracheal tube (ETT). We have found it easier in children requiring intubation with a 4.5-mm ETT or less to place the bronchial blocker outside of the ETT to avoid decreasing the lumen of the ETT and improve ventilation of the single lung. This can be achieved by first intubating the trachea with an appropriate-size tube, placing the bronchial blocker with fiberoptic guidance through the ETT, removing the initial ETT, and then intubating alongside the bronchial blocker. Always check the position of the ETT and the blocker with a fiberoptic bronchoscope, and recheck it in the lateral position. It is much harder to provide a good seal when placing a blocker down the right side because of the acute takeoff of the right upper lobe bronchus.

POSTOPERATIVE CONSIDERATIONS

Extubation of the trachea at the conclusion of the case should be planned, especially if a thoroscopic approach was used. Postoperative pain management needs to be addressed and is especially important after an open thoracotomy, since there may be pleural and muscle damage, possible disruption of the costovertebral joint, and intercostal nerve damage secondary to the surgery. One can consider a thoracic epidural that is placed preincision with its position verified using fluoroscopy, a paravertebral extrapleural catheter placed under direct visualization, or a pleural catheter. Because of the increased risk of placing a thoracic epidural in an anesthetized patient, one can consider placing a caudal catheter and inserting an epidural catheter up to the desired thoracic level with fluoroscopy or stimulation guidance. In adult patients, a paravertebral extrapleural catheter is as efficacious as a thoracic epidural and has fewer complications. Information about local anesthetic uptake from either the extrapleural or pleural space in the pediatric population is sparse, but existing data suggest a rapid uptake of the local anesthetic; thus, local anesthetic toxicity must be considered when choosing the appropriate drug.

DOs and DON'Ts

✓ Do provide lung isolation to facilitate thoracoscopic surgery (Table 23-1).
✓ Do confirm the perfect position of the ETT before bringing the patient into the lateral position. Once the patient is in the lateral position, it becomes very cumbersome to manipulate the ETT.
✓ Do remember that the simplest way to isolate the lung in small infants is to simply advance the ETT in the mainstem. This is the most straightforward solution, since bronchial blockers need constant adjustments throughout the case.

(Continue)

✓ Use 100% oxygen shortly before lung separation to increase absorption and better collapse of the operative side.
✓ Humidify airway gases to prevent heat loss and concretion of pulmonary secretions.
✓ Provide postoperative pain control, especially if an open thoracotomy approach is utilized.

SURGICAL CONCERNS

Early surgical intervention resolves respiratory distress seen in the infant, prevents recurrent infections, and helps spare normal tissue.

FACTOID

Sequestration of the lung represents about 6% of all congenital pulmonary malformations. The most common location of the sequestered lung is in the posterior basal segment, with nearly two-thirds in the left lung. An intrapulmonary sequestration may be asymptomatic and not be discovered until adulthood. Extrapulmonary sequestrations can be found in unexpected places (for example, the diaphragm or mediastinum).

TABLE 23-1   SIZE CHART FOR LUNG SEPARATION

Age (years)	ETT (interior diameter in mm)	BB (Fr)	Univent	DLT (Fr)
0.5-1	3.5-4.0	5		
1-2	4.0-4.5	5		
2-4	4.5-5.0	5		
4-6	5.0-5.0 cuffed	5		
6-8	5.5 cuffed	5	3.5	
8-10	6.0 cuffed	5	3.5	26
10-12	6.5 cuffed	5	4.5	26-28
12-14	6.5-7.0 cuffed	5 or 7	4.5	32
14-16	7.0 cuffed	7 or 9	6.0	35
16-18	8.0 cuffed	7 or 9	7.0	35

BB: bronchial blocker 5-9 (Arnt bronchial blocker, Cook Incorporated, Bloomington, IN, USA).
DLT: double lumen tube 26-35 (RUSCH, Teleflex Medical, Athlone, Ireland).
ETT: endotracheal tube 3.5-8.0 (Portex tracheal tubes, Smiths Medical ASD, Keene, NH, USA).
Table adapted from Hammer G. "Single Lung Ventilation in Infants and Children." *Pediatr Anesth.* 2004;14:98-102.

PART 4

NEONATES

24 NECROTIZING ENTEROCOLITIS

Neeta R. Saraiya, MD

YOUR PATIENT

A 1.5-kg, 28-week premature neonate develops abdominal distention and bloody stool after first feedings. Patient appears lethargic with increasing respiratory effort.

Laboratory: Hematocrit (Hct) 25; platelets 50,000; blood gas: pH 7.2, CO_2 65, BE10, HCO_3 18.
Abdominal x-ray: Free air with bowel distention.

PREOPERATIVE CONSIDERATIONS

Necrotizing enterocolitis (NEC) affects 1-7% of patients admitted to the neonatal intensive care unit. It's a life-threatening intestinal inflammation where the injury is caused by reduced mesenteric blood flow. Mortality due to NEC is 55%. Risk factors are multifactorial prematurity, although cardiac and pulmonary diseases play a major role.

Patients present with increased gastric residuals with feeding, abdominal distention, bilious vomiting, lethargy, fever or hypothermia, and gross or occult rectal bleeding. Abdominal x-rays show distended loops of bowel, pneumatosis intestinalis, and air in the portal vein or pneumoperitoneum. The complete blood cell count and electrolytes may be altered, and the patient may develop disseminated intravascular coagulation (DIC).

Medical management is attempted first, with the patient being given nothing by mouth, and antibiotics, hemodynamic support, and transfusion as needed. If there is evidence of free air, patients may need to have surgery.

ANESTHETIC MANAGEMENT

- If patient is not intubated, then take full stomach precautions; do rapid-sequence induction or awake intubation.
- Continuous and aggressive fluid resuscitation may require up to 100 mL/kg.
- Prevention of hypothermia is required.

- Inotropic agents should be given if needed for cardiovascular support.
- Transfusion of fresh frozen plasma, red blood cells, and platelets may be needed, since patients may present with DIC.
- An opioid-based anesthetic is best tolerated.

POSTOPERATIVE CONSIDERATIONS

Postoperative ventilation is required. Patients may come back to the operating room 24-48 hours later for a second look exploration. Long-term complications may include intestinal strictures and short gut syndrome.

DOs and DON'Ts

✓   Do awake or rapid-sequence induction.
⊗   Do not start the case without having blood products immediately available.
✓   Do prevent hypothermia.

SURGICAL CONCERNS

Exploratory laparotomy with resection of the necrotic segment of the intestine and an ileostomy is performed. If the infant is <1000 g and hemodynamically unstable, a bedside percutaneous intraperitoneal drain is placed.

FACTOID

NEC is rarely seen in full-term neonates. It continues to be a significant cause of mortality and morbidity in preterm patients. Even with aggressive medical management and timely surgical intervention, the mortality remains >50%.

25 PYLORIC STENOSIS

Philipp J. Houck, MD

YOUR PATIENT

A 6-week-old child presents with a history of intolerance to feedings. The patient has had nonbilious projectile vomiting for the past 48 hours, vomiting immediately after feedings.

Laboratory: K 5.9; HCO_3 30; Cl 96 (after 24 hours of hydration, K 4.7; HCO_3 23; Cl 101).

Physical exam: Olive-shaped mass palpated in right upper quadrant.

PREOPERATIVE CONSIDERATIONS

Pyloric stenosis is a hypertrophy of the pyloric muscles, typically seen between 2 and 12 weeks of age. Patients present with projectile vomiting after feedings, dehydration, and failure to thrive. The diagnosis can be made by history and physical examination alone; barium swallow and ultrasound are confirmatory tests. Ongoing loss of potassium, hydrogen, and chloride ions leads to contraction alkalosis. The loss of potassium through vomiting, the exchange of hydrogen ions for extracellular potassium, and the renal potassium loss all lead to hypokalemia.

The patient should have a plasma chloride >100 and urine chloride >20; serum bicarbonate should be less than 28 mEq/dL prior to the surgery.

Once diagnosed, patients should be given nothing by mouth, a nasogastric tube should be inserted, and intravenous fluids should be administered. Pyloric stenosis is not a surgical, but a medical emergency.

ANESTHETIC MANAGEMENT

- Decompress the stomach prior to initiating induction. Consider using an anticholinergic to blunt the vagal response to suctioning. Consider sitting the patient upright and rolling the patient from side to side to ensure that all gastric content is aspirated.
- Consider awake intubation versus rapid-sequence induction.
- Be cautious when using muscle relaxant; large doses of rocuronium can last for hours.

- Avoid opioids; rectal acetaminophen and infiltration with local anesthetic are sufficient.
- Maintain anesthesia with sevoflurane or desflurane and a remifentanil infusion. You may give a small amount of a muscle relaxant for the incision and then limit the volatile anesthetic.

POSTOPERATIVE CONSIDERATIONS

Most patients can start feeding within hours. No intensive care unit admission is necessary.

DOs and DON'Ts

✓ Do an awake intubation, a rapid-sequence induction, or a modified rapid-sequence induction.

⊗ Do not do a mask induction.

✓ Do empty the stomach with the patient in four different positions prior to airway management.

⊗ Do not give opioids.

CONTROVERSIES

- Awake intubation vs rapid-sequence induction
- Succinylcholine vs nondepolarizing muscle relaxants

SURGICAL CONCERNS

Mucosal damage was initially reported more often with the laparoscopic approach. A leak can be detected intraoperatively by inflating the stomach with an orogastric tube; the pylorus is observed for leaking air.

FACTOID

In developing countries, pyloric stenosis is treated mainly with medical management, which includes anticholinergics and fluid management for two weeks. Only patients who medically failed (20%!) are operated on.

26 CONGENITAL DIAPHRAGMATIC HERNIA

Neeta R. Saraiya, MD

YOUR PATIENT

A full-term infant born with Apgars of 6, 5, and 5 with severe respiratory distress and a weak cry appears dyspneic and cyanotic.

> *Physical examination*: The baby has a barrel-shaped chest and scaphoid abdomen. Upon auscultation, there are decreased breath sounds, and bowel sounds can be heard in the left chest.
>
> *Chest x-ray*: Mediastinum is pushed to the right and air-filled loops of bowel are present in the left chest.

PREOPERATIVE CONSIDERATIONS

Congenital diaphragmatic hernia (CDH) occurs due to in utero herniation of abdominal contents into the thoracic cavity through a defect in the diaphragm, most commonly (80%) via the left pleuroperitoneal canal (foramen of Bochdalek). As a result, the hemithorax is filled with stomach and intestine. The herniated bowel prevents normal lung development on the ipsilateral side. The contralateral lung is also affected, with reduced-size bronchi, less bronchial branching, decreased alveolar surface area, and abnormal pulmonary vasculature characterized by thickening of arteriolar smooth muscle. Less commonly, the defect can be in the anterior diaphragm (Morgani, retrosternal, or parasternal hernia). This occurs more commonly on the right side.

Incidence is 1 in 2500 live births, with 44-66% having other congenital anomalies, including 4-16% with chromosomal anomalies.

In the past decade, medical stabilization of the patient has come to be done prior to surgical repair. Management is directed toward reducing pulmonary hypertension with nitric oxide, moderate alkalosis, and permissive hypercapnia. Patients who are unable to tolerate conventional ventilation are placed on high-frequency oscillatory ventilation. Patients who have failed medical management may be placed on extracorporeal membrane oxygenation (ECMO).

ANESTHETIC MANAGEMENT

- Patients are intubated in the neonatal intensive care unit immediately after birth.
- Be careful with positive pressure ventilation so as to not overinflate the healthy lung.
- Maintenance is done with volatile agents plus IV narcotics plus muscle relaxant.
- Avoid nitrous oxide.
- Avoid an increase in pulmonary vascular resistance (PVR) leading to right-to-left shunting, eg, hypoxia, acidosis, hypothermia, and pain.
- Mild permissive hypercapnia is usually well tolerated (pCO_2 50-60).
- Replace significant blood loss.

POSTOPERATIVE CONSIDERATIONS

Postoperatively, these patients continue to require ventilatory support. There may be worsening of pulmonary hypertension and clinical deterioration despite surgical repair. If sudden deterioration of clinical status occurs, consider pneumothorax on the contralateral side.

DOs and DON'Ts

- ⊗ Do not mask ventilate.
- ⊗ Do not attempt to manually inflate the contralateral lung; it is at risk for pneumothorax.
- ⊗ Do not use nitrous oxide.
- ✓ Do use pressure-limited ventilation to maintain preductal oxygen saturation at greater than 85-90%; tolerate mild hypercapnia.

SURGICAL REPAIR

Surgical repair is via a subcostal transabdominal incision on the affected side. The bowel is reduced from the chest, and the diaphragmatic defect is repaired either by primary closure or by Gore-Tex patch.

Attempts have been made to do thoracoscopic repair of CDH. Because of the high incidence of recurrence of CDH after the repair, this approach has lost some supporters.

FACTOID

Survival rates of 50-60% with ECMO have been reported in selected patients in whom a 90% mortality is expected.

27 TRACHEOESOPHAGEAL FISTULA

Neeta R. Saraiya, MD

YOUR PATIENT

A 38-week-gestation male child who was born with Apgars of 8 and 9 is unable to pass the nasogastric tube. The patient starts coughing and choking with pooling of secretions in the mouth. He is unable to swallow.

Chest x-ray shows the nasogastric tube coiled up in the chest and a big gastric bubble.

Physical examination shows bilateral equal breath sounds with a distended abdomen and systolic murmur.

PREOPERATIVE CONSIDERATIONS

The incidence of tracheoesophageal fistula (TEF) is 1 in 3000-4500 live births, and 35-65% of patients have associated congenital anomalies. This anomaly may be part of the VACTERL (vertebral anomalies, anorectal malformation, cardiac anomalies, tracheoesophageal fistula, esophageal atresia, renal anomalies, and limb anomalies) association. There are different types of TEF with varying incidence, with the commonest type being type C. Patients present with the "3Cs of esophageal atresia" (choking, coughing, and cyanosis) because of an inability to swallow and may develop aspiration pneumonia.

Patients should have a chest x-ray, echocardiography to rule out any cardiac anomaly, and a complete blood cell count and serum electrolytes to rule out renal anomalies.

Once diagnosed, the patient is given nothing by mouth, and a nasogastric tube is placed in the upper pouch with suction in the head up position. Antibiotics are started. Surgery is performed after 24-48 hours of stabilization.

ANESTHETIC MANAGEMENT

- In premature patients with a cardiac lesion, consider staged repair, with placement of a gastrostomy tube under local or spinal anesthesia, subsequent ligation of the fistula, and esophageal repair when stable.

- Use IV and/or inhalation induction until the airway is secure and adequate ventilation is assured.
- The goal is to place the tip of the endotracheal tube beyond the origin of the fistula.
- Avoid controlled ventilation; spontaneous and gently assisted ventilation is preferred until the fistula is ligated.
- A good option is to maintain anesthesia with sevoflurane and remifentanil infusion.
- Constant communication with the surgeon is crucial.

POSTOPERATIVE CONSIDERATIONS

The goal should be to return to spontaneous ventilation and extubation as soon as possible to avoid ventilation in a patient with a fresh tracheal anastomosis. These patients are at risk of developing tracheomalacia, mediastinitis, and sepsis due to leakage from the site of the esophageal anastomosis. Usually there is some residual esophageal dysfunction, decreased esophageal motility, and stricture formation.

DOs and DON'Ts

✓ Do IV and/or inhalation induction with spontaneous ventilation.
⊗ Do not give positive pressure ventilation.
⊗ Do not give muscle relaxant until the surgeon has control of the fistula.

SURGICAL MANAGEMENT

A retropleural approach via a right thoracotomy with the child in left lateral decubitis position is commonly used. The new trend is toward thoracoscopic repair of TEF, where thoracoscopy introduces significant physiologic changes: right-sided thoracoscopy reduces venous return and mean arterial blood pressure, and CO_2 absorption causes hypercarbia and acidosis, which can lead to increased pulmonary vascular resistance (PVR). PVR is dependent on $PaCO_2$, PaO_2, pH, and lung volumes.

FACTOID

Prognosis of patients with TEF is primarily dependent on the presence of prematurity and other congenital anomalies. Coexisting major congenital heart disease and low birth weight <1500 g can reduce survival from 97%-99% to 22%-43%.

28 GASTROSCHISIS AND OMPHALOCELE

Neeta R. Saraiya, MD

YOUR PATIENT

A male child born via cesarean section at 35 weeks' gestation presents with protrusion of bowel outside the abdominal cavity.

The patient was prenatally diagnosed with an abdominal wall defect.

Physical examination shows an alert, awake baby with protrusion of the small intestine outside the abdomen with no peritoneal covering.

PREOPERATIVE CONSIDERATIONS

Major defects in closure of the abdominal wall result in exposure of the viscera. In *omphalocele*, the viscera herniate through the umbilicus and are covered with the peritoneum. In *gastroschisis*, the viscera herniate through a defect lateral to the umbilicus, usually to the right, and have no covering.

The incidence is 1 in 6000-10 000 live births for omphalocele and 1 in 30 000 live births for gastroschisis. About two-thirds of patients with omphalocele have associated congenital anomalies, such as cardiovascular, genitourinary, gastrointestinal, or craniofacial anomalies, trisomy 13, or Beckwith-Wiedemann syndrome (visceromegaly, macroglossia, microcephaly, and hypoglycemia).

These patients are cared for expeditiously to minimize the potential for heat loss from the exposed viscera, minimize the possibility of infection, and prevent direct trauma to the herniated organs. The stomach is decompressed with a nasogastric tube, and broad-spectrum antibiotics are initiated.

Aggressive fluid resuscitation with a balanced salt solution (150-300 mL/kg/d) is initiated to maintain urine output at 1-2 mL/kg/h.

ANESTHETIC MANAGEMENT

- Prior to induction, suction the stomach.
- Use preoxygenation.
- Use either awake intubation or rapid-sequence induction with endotracheal intubation.
- Ensure adequate fluid resuscitation with a balanced salt solution.

- Prevent hypothermia.
- Maintain with a narcotic-based anesthetic and a nondepolarizing muscle relaxant.

POSTOPERATIVE CONSIDERATIONS

Patients require postoperative ventilation with fluid resuscitation along with broad-spectrum antibiotics. Patients are at risk of developing abdominal compartment syndrome if the abdominal closure is too tight.

Criteria used as guidelines to monitor intraabdominal pressure are intragastric pressure <20 cm H_2O, intravesical pressure <20 cm H_2O, and maximum peak ventilatory pressure <30 cm H_2O.

DOs and DON'Ts

✓   Do obtain a preoperative echocardiogram in patients with omphalocele.
⊗   Do not mask ventilate the patient.
✓   Do aggressive fluid resuscitation.
✓   Do communicate with the surgeon if abdominal closure is too tight.
✓   Do give adequate nondepolarizing muscle relaxant to facilitate abdominal closure.

SURGICAL CONCERNS

The goal is to place the exposed viscera into the abdomen. If the defect is small, primary complete closure is attempted. If a large amount of viscera is exposed, then a staged closure with a silastic silo is performed; the silo is secured at the edge of the defect and gradually reduced over 3-7 days. The patient is then brought to the operating room for complete closure.

FACTOID

Premature labor and delivery is common with gastroschisis, possibly because of irritation of the exposed small bowel. The incidence of other associated congenital anomalies is lower in patients with gastroschisis, but they tend to have more issues with bowel function. Congenital heart disease significantly increases mortality in patients with omphalocele.

29 DUODENAL ATRESIA

Neeta R. Saraiya, MD

YOUR PATIENT

A 1-day-old child with trisomy 21 born after 32 weeks' gestation presents with bilious vomiting. Prenatal ultrasound was significant for polyhydramnios.

An abdominal x-ray shows a dilated stomach, a dilated first part of the duodenum (double bubble), and absence of air beyond the second air bubble.

PREOPERATIVE CONSIDERATIONS

Duodenal atresia results from failure to recanalize the lumen of the duodenum after the solid phase of embryologic development. Between 38% and 55% of patients with duodenal atresia have another associated significant congenital anomaly: approximately 30% of cases are associated with Down syndrome, and 23%-34% of cases are associated with isolated cardiac defects. Esophageal atresia may be present in 7%-12% of patients. Other gastrointestinal anomalies include malrotation, anorectal anomalies, intestinal atresias, cloacal anomalies, annular pancreas, and renal anomalies. Duodenal atresia is associated with prematurity and low birth weight. Duodenal atresia is prenatally detected in 32%-57% of patients, and fetal ultrasound may show polyhydramnios.

Patients present with vomiting, which can be bilious or nonbilious. The abdominal x-ray shows a "double bubble." Once diagnosed, patients are given nothing by mouth, a nasogastric tube is inserted, and intravenous fluids are started.

ANESTHETIC CONSIDERATIONS

- Decompress the stomach.
- Use preoxygenation and intravenous atropine 10 μg/kg.
- Use either awake intubation or rapid-sequence IV induction with endotracheal intubation.
- Avoid hypothermia.

- Maintain anesthesia with sevoflurane or narcotics and muscle relaxants.
- Fluid replacement for the third space and insensible fluid loss is needed in addition to the maintenance fluid requirements.

POSTOPERATIVE CONSIDERATIONS

Postoperative complications are reported in 14%-18% of patients. Possible indications for reoperation include anastomotic leak, functional duodenal obstruction, adhesions, and missed atresias.

The patients are given nothing by mouth until bowel sounds are heard, stool is passed, and the gastric drainage is limited (<1 mL/kg/h of clear or pale-green fluid). This may take 7-10 days, but it can be prolonged in the premature infant with other significant anomalies and may require intravenous total parental nutrition.

DOs and DON'Ts

⊗   Do not mask ventilate.
✓   Do decompress the stomach prior to induction.

SURGICAL CONCERNS

The operative management of duodenal atresia is determined by the anatomic findings and associated anomalies noted upon laparotomy. Bypass procedures for duodenal atresia or stenosis include duodenoduodenostomy and duodenojejunostomy.

FACTOID

Current survival rates for infants with duodenal atresia or stenosis are 90%-95%. Higher mortality rates are associated with prematurity and multiple congenital abnormalities.

30 MALROTATION

Neeta R. Saraiya, MD

YOUR PATIENT

A 3-week-old full-term infant born with hypoplastic left heart syndrome presents with bilious vomiting for 2 days. The patient appears irritable.

Laboratory: HCO_3 20; BE 8; hematocrit (Hct) 30

An upper GI contrast study shows duodenojejunal flexure to the right of the midline, jejunal loops on the right side of the abdomen, and a high cecum on delayed film.

PREOPERATIVE CONSIDERATIONS

Intestinal malrotation is a developmental anomaly that affects the position and peritoneal attachments of the small and large intestines during organogenesis in fetal life. Intestinal malrotation occurs in 1 in 500 live births. Male predominance is present during neonatal presentations, with a male-to-female ratio of 2:1. About 40% of patients with malrotation present within the first week of life, 50% at up to 1 month of age, and 75% by the age of 1 year; the remaining 25% present later, even into adult life.

Malrotation may be associated with other congenital abnormalities, including congenital heart disease, diaphragmatic hernia, esophageal atresia, duodenal or jejunal web or atresia, omphalocele, and gastroschisis.

Patients either are diagnosed as an incidental finding and will present to the operating room for an elective Ladd's procedure or will present with a tender, distended abdomen and bilious vomiting secondary to bowel obstruction. Acidosis due to dehydration and bowel ischemia is associated with volvulus.

If malrotation is associated with volvulus, it is an absolute surgical emergency.

ANESTHETIC MANAGEMENT

- When this is an elective procedure, mask or IV induction is acceptable.
- Full stomach precautions should be taken during induction if the patient is obstructed, including rapid-sequence IV induction.

- Consider an arterial line if the patient is obstructed or has a congenital cardiac disease.
- Aggressive fluid resuscitation with large volumes of colloids and blood and circulatory support with pressors may be needed.
- Correction of acidosis is done initially with fluid resuscitation followed with bicarbonate, diluted to 0.5 mEq/mL to avoid causing acute hypernatremia, which could increase the risk of intracerebral bleeding in neonates.
- Opioid-based anesthetics are best tolerated.
- Patients with associated congenital cardiac disease, especially those with Blalock-Taussig shunts, have to be aggressively fluid resuscitated to avoid clotting of their shunts.

POSTOPERATIVE CONSIDERATIONS

Patients may require admission to the intensive care unit if this condition is associated with other congenital anomalies. Patients may require postoperative fluid resuscitation. Risk of postoperative bowel obstruction does exist after Ladd's procedure.

DOs and DON'Ts

✓   Do use rapid-sequence induction when patients are obstructed.
✓   Do aggressive fluid resuscitation and replacement of the third space extracellular fluid loss.

SURGICAL MANAGEMENT

The surgical management of malrotation is based on Ladd's procedure. The base of the mesenteric pedicle is broadened by dividing the peritoneal bands that tether the small bowel and colon to the mesentery. Ladd's peritoneal bands are completely divided, and an appendectomy is performed.

FACTOID

The incidence of malrotation is higher in patients with heterotaxia. Patients with heterotaxia and malrotation have better outcomes if they have an elective Ladd's procedure after correction or palliation of the cardiac anomaly.

31 MECONIUM ILEUS

Leila M. Pang, MD

YOUR PATIENT

A 3.1-kg 1-day-old male born at term is scheduled for an exploratory laparotomy for meconium ileus.

Vital signs: BP = 55/35; P = 130
Laboratory: Hematocrit (Hct) = 45%

PREOPERATIVE CONSIDERATIONS

Meconium ileus is seen soon after birth when an infant with a distended abdomen fails to pass meconium. It is often possible to palpate a mass in the right lower quadrant that corresponds to the distended ileum obstructed by the abnormal meconium. Perforation may occur in utero. When this occurs, meconium peritonitis with calcification follows and may be visualized radiographically. This may lead to atresia or stenosis of the bowel segment, volvulus, and necrosis. The cause is the presence of abnormally viscid meconium with an increased protein content that cannot be propelled by the bowel. When a single or multiple ileal atresias are present in the newborn or meconium ileus is found, the diagnosis of cystic fibrosis should be suspected. Respiratory symptoms of cystic fibrosis are generally not present in the neonatal period.

Intestinal anomalies other than ileal atresia are rarely associated with meconium ileus.

ANESTHETIC MANAGEMENT

- Two peripheral IVs.
- Consider an arterial line. Monitoring acid-base status and hematocrit may be helpful in guiding fluid resuscitation.
- Rapid-sequence induction vs awake intubation—consider providing oxygen during laryngoscopy to delay or decrease the amount of desaturation that may occur.
- Use narcotics judiciously if planning extubation.
- Warm forced air and fluid.

POSTOPERATIVE CONSIDERATIONS

Extubation of the trachea at the conclusion of the case should be entertained.

DOs and DON'Ts

✓   Do aggressively maintain fluid volume, as large amounts of fluid may be lost as evaporative and third space losses.
✓   Do warm the patient aggressively, since a significant portion of the patient's body surface area may be exposed.

SURGICAL CONCERNS

If surgical evacuation of the meconium is unsuccessful, an enterostomy will need to be created.

FACTOID

Meconium ileus is found almost exclusively in patients with cystic fibrosis. However, only about 20% of the patients with cystic fibrosis will have meconium ileus.

32 IMPERFORATE ANUS

Leila M. Pang, MD

YOUR PATIENT

A 2-day-old male newborn has not passed any meconium since birth. Examination of the newborn reveals no anal orifice. The newborn is scheduled for a colostomy.

PREOPERATIVE CONSIDERATIONS

An imperforate anus may occur with several presentations.

Type 1: Anal stenosis occurs at the anus or 1-4 cm above the anal level and is due to the incomplete rupture of the anal membrane. There may be an associated fistula with the genitourinary system or the perineum.

Type 2: Imperforate anus occurs when the obstruction is due to a persistent membrane.

Type 3 (the most common presentation): Imperforate anus is associated with the rectum ending blindly at a considerable distance above the imperforate anus. The rectum may have a fistulous connection to the urethra, bladder, base of the penis or scrotum, or vagina.

Type 4: There is a normal anus and anal pouch, but the rectum ends blindly.

The newborn may present because no stool has been passed in the first 24 hours, because the newborn has a distended abdomen, or because the newborn passes stool near the vaginal opening, the base of the scrotum, the bladder, or the penis.

Imperforate anus may also occur with other congenital abnormalities, such as VACTERL (vertebral, anal, cardiac, tracheal, esophageal, renal, and limb) and REAR (renal, ear, anal, and radial) syndromes. In general, the higher the anorectal anomaly is located, the greater the incidence of associated anomalies. The incidence of anorectal malformations is about 1 in 5000 newborns.

The newborn should be screened for associated abnormalities preoperatively, especially for cardiac and tracheoesophageal anomalies.

ANESTHETIC MANAGEMENT

- Anesthesia should be adapted to the extent of the abdominal distention, the operation (simple perineal anoplasty, temporary colostomy, or extensive abdominoperineal repair), and whether there are any associated cardiovascular and renal problems.
- Consider rapid-sequence induction or awake intubation if the abdomen is distended.
- Maintain anesthesia with an inhalational agent in an air-oxygen mixture. Use muscle relaxants to allow better operating conditions. If there is no need to identify the anal sphincter. Use narcotics judiciously.
- Nitrous oxide should be avoided to prevent further bowel distention.
- Ensure adequate hydration, as there may be large insensible fluid losses, large third space losses with bowel manipulation, and additional considerations if there is a bowel perforation. Balanced salt solutions or colloid at a rate of 10 mL/kg/h of surgery or more may be needed.
- Consider the risk of sepsis if there was bowel perforation.
- Monitoring includes urine output, blood pressure, and quality of heart tones. Invasive monitoring is not required for the healthy patient.

POSTOPERATIVE CONSIDERATIONS

If there are other associated life-threatening anomalies or if a large volume of fluids was required to keep the patient hemodynamically stable, you should consider keeping the patient intubated and ventilated at the end of the case.

DOs and DON'Ts

✓   Do consider a rapid-sequence or modified rapid-sequence induction or an awake intubation.
✓   Do keep up with blood and fluid losses.
✓   Do adapt your technique to take into consideration any associated cardiac and/or renal problems.
⊗   Do not use nitrous oxide, as this may further distend the bowel.

CONTROVERSIES

Awake intubation vs rapid-sequence induction
Succinylcholine vs nondepolarizing muscle relaxants for intubation

SURGICAL CONCERNS

For an extensive abdominoperineal repair, the surgeon may need to identify the anal sphincter by using direct muscle stimulation; thus, large doses of nondepolarizing muscle relaxants that create profound muscle relaxation may not be a good idea.

FACTOID

In a review of 25 years of experience dealing with children with anorectal abnormalities, there was a 20% overall mortality rate, with the greatest number of these patients having a high type 3 lesion. Approximately 80% of these deaths were unrelated to the imperforate anus but resulted from the associated anomalies. About 88 % of the surviving patients were able to achieve socially acceptable continence.

33 MYELOMENINGOCELE

Leila M. Pang, MD

YOUR PATIENT

A 1-day-old male newborn is scheduled for a repair of a meningo-myelocele. At the time of birth, examination of the newborn revealed a lumbosacral defect that was partially epithelialized. The defect was covered with a sterile dressing, and the child was placed in a partial lateral decubitus position.

PREOPERATIVE CONSIDERATIONS

The meningomyelocele may occur with several presentations. Most commonly, fusion of the neural tube fails in the middle or caudal neural groove, resulting in a thoracic or lumbosacral meningomyelocele. When the site of failed closure occurs more cephalad, encephaloceles result. The defective neural tissue in meningomyeloceles is in open communication with the environment; thus, an early closure to minimize bacterial contamination is recommended.

There can be an association with hydrocephalus and Chiari malformation. Most congenital lesions of the central nervous system (CNS) are not associated with an increased incidence of anomalies of other organ systems.

The incidence of meningomyelocele is about 1-6 in every 1000 live births.

ANESTHETIC MANAGEMENT

- Positioning for induction and intubation in order to avoid physical trauma to the neuroplaque may be a challenge. The patient should be supported by portions of the back that are not involved using rolled towels or a "doughnut" ring cushion.
- Inhalational or IV induction may be used.
- Maintenance of anesthesia is done with an inhalational agent in an air-oxygen mixture. Muscle relaxants may be used if the surgeon does not expect to use a nerve stimulator. Use narcotics judiciously.
- Succinylcholine is not associated with excessive hyperkalemia in these patients.

- Monitoring includes urine output and temperature. Invasive monitoring is not required for the healthy patient.
- Conservation of body heat is important, since autonomic control below the defect is usually impaired.
- Blood loss is usually small, but it may increase if the surgeon has to undermine a large area of skin and fascia to achieve primary closure.
- Keep up with ongoing insensible fluid losses.

POSTOPERATIVE CONSIDERATIONS

You may consider keeping the patient intubated and ventilated at the end of the case because of the age of the patient and the potential association with the Chiari malformation, which can be associated with an abnormal ventilatory response to hypoxia.

DOs and DON'Ts

✓ Do carefully position the patient for induction and intubation.
✓ Do conserve body heat.
✓ Do keep up with insensible fluid losses.

CONTROVERSIES

A ventriculoperitoneal shunt can be placed at the time of initial closure of the meningomyelocele, but some surgeons prefer waiting for a few days, especially in patients without apparent hydrocephalus at birth.

SURGICAL CONCERNS

For lumbosacral repair, the surgeon may want to use direct muscle stimulation to spare neurological tissue; thus, large doses of nondepolarizing muscle relaxants that create profound muscle relaxation may not be a good idea.

FACTOID

Myelodysplasia (including meningomyelocele) is caused by a congenital failure of the neural tube to close. This process usually occurs by 28 days of gestation. Neurological function is frequently severely impaired caudal to the defect. There has been a decrease in these malformations since the promotion of ingestion of folic acid before and during the first 3 months of pregnancy.

34 SACROCOCCYGEAL TUMOR

Leila M. Pang, MD

YOUR PATIENT

A 2.8-kg 2-day-old male born at 33 weeks' gestation is scheduled for elective resection of a very large sacrococcygeal teratoma. He is on room air with nasal continuous positive airway pressure (CPAP).

Vital signs: BP = 55/35, P = 150
Laboratory: Hematocrit (Hct) = 45%

PREOPERATIVE CONSIDERATIONS

Sacrococcygeal teratoma is the most common tumor of the newborn, occurring in 1 in 35000-40000 live births. It occurs more often in females, with a 3-4:1 ratio. Often the tumor is small and presents as a lump in the sacral region.

This tumor can present prenatally secondary to the abnormal size of the uterus for the calculated gestational age of the fetus and can even outgrow the fetus in size. It can be associated with fetal hydrops leading to polyhydramnios and premature delivery or can rapidly progress to fatality in utero secondary to the high-output cardiac failure resulting from the "vascular steal" of blood flow through the tumor. Maternal symptoms may mimic the fetal symptoms, also jeopardizing maternal health.

ANESTHETIC MANAGEMENT

- If the tumor is large, positioning may be difficult, and creative padding may be required to allow the patient to lie supine without distortion from the tumor.
- Use standard American Society of Anesthesiologists monitors with two IVs and an arterial line, and consider central venous pressure monitoring if the tumor is large.
- Use IV or inhalational induction.
- Consider IV or inhalational maintenance with short-acting opioids such as remifentanil or fentanyl.
- Avoid hypothermia in such small patients by using a forced warm air device, and consider using a fluid warmer.

POSTOPERATIVE CONSIDERATIONS

Extubation at the conclusion of the case is probably not a good idea, since these patients tend to be premature and have a high incidence of apnea and bradycardia in the postoperative period. In addition, the patient may need to be maintained in the prone position, so airway access may be more difficult in an emergency situation.

DOs and DON'Ts

✓ Do aggressively maintain fluid volume, as large amounts of fluid may be lost evaporatively.

✓ Do warm the patient aggressively, since a significant portion of the patient's body surface area may be exposed.

⊗ Do not extubate at the end of the case, especially if the patient is premature.

FACTOID

The majority of these neonatal tumors are benign, so the prognosis after surgery is excellent.

PART 5

NEURO

35 HYDROCEPHALUS

Leila M. Pang, MD

YOUR PATIENT

A 3-month-old, former 33-week-gestation premature, male infant presents with a history of increasing irritability and lethargy and vomiting of 2 days' duration. The infant has a history of a grade III intraventricular hemorrhage in the newborn period that required a ventriculoperitoneal (VP) shunt. The neurologist and neurosurgeons have already obtained an x-ray and have determined that the existing VP shunt is blocked. He is scheduled for an emergency VP shunt revision.

PREOPERATIVE CONSIDERATIONS

Hydrocephalus is not a disease in itself but a consequence of a disease process. In the neonatal period, the most common causes for hydrocephalus are anatomic anomalies associated with myelodysplasia and prematurity (intraventricular hemorrhage). Other causes include obstruction or a mass effect caused by tumors or a decrease in cerebrospinal fluid resorption secondary to scar or fibrin deposition postcraniotomy. Patients present with bulging fontanelles and ophthalmoplegia (in the newborn period), headaches, irritability, lethargy, and vomiting. This can progress to seizures and finally to herniation of the brain stem.

The presence or absence of increased intracranial pressure (ICP) must be assessed prior to induction. If increased ICP is present, no premedication should be given. Other factors to consider should be pulmonary status (especially if the patient is a former premature infant), seizure history and medications, and physical limitations.

ANESTHETIC MANAGEMENT

- In patients with longstanding hydrocephalus, the head circumference will be increased. Accessing the oral cavity with the laryngoscope may be challenging if the occiput causes extreme flexion of the head, so consider elevating the patient's shoulders and/or torso to put the head in a neutral position.
- Induce anesthesia via IV or inhalation, if a full stomach is not a consideration.

- If the patient has not been fasted appropriately or is vomiting, then consider a rapid-sequence induction using a nondepolarizing muscle relaxant such as rocuronium (1 mg/kg IV) rather than a depolarizing muscle relaxant to prevent an increase in gastric pressure and vomiting and an increase in intracranial pressure. The use of a depolarizing muscle relaxant is not absolutely contraindicated and should be considered if the need for immediate control of the airway outweighs the risks of a transient increase in intracranial pressure.
- In the premature infant especially, use the lowest possible fraction of inspired oxygen (FiO_2) needed to maintain oxygen saturations above 90% to minimize the risk of retinopathy of prematurity.
- Avoid hypercapnia and a halogenated agent, especially in the patient with an elevated ICP, until the cranium is opened.
- Consider using an intravenous anesthetic rather than an inhalational anesthetic to avoid vasodilation.

POSTOPERATIVE CONSIDERATIONS

The premature and former premature infant is at risk for postoperative apneic episodes for a period lasting up to 60 weeks postconception and should have cardiorespiratory monitoring for 24 hours postoperatively.

DOs and DON'Ts

✓ Do maintain normocapnia or mild hypocapnia (end-tidal CO_2 [$EtCO_2$] ≈ 30-35 mm Hg) until the cranium is open to help maintain cerebral perfusion pressure and prevent further increasing the elevated ICP.

✓ Avoid hypotension to prevent the risk of decreasing cerebral perfusion pressure.

✓ Do cardiopulmonary monitoring postoperatively in the premature and former premature infant who is at risk for postoperative apnea.

⊗ Do not use a halogenated agent until the cranium is open to help control the increased ICP.

⊗ Do not use a depolarizing muscle relaxant that will increase ICP, unless warranted.

CONTROVERSIES

Do not overhyperventilate, but rather maintain normocapnia or a mild hypocapnia to prevent an increase in intracranial pressure.

SURGICAL CONCERNS

There is a higher incidence of VP shunt revisions in patients who had the initial VP shunt placed before the age of 6 months. Among all patients, up to 16% require a revision within a month and up to 40% within a year. The most common risk factor is a patient characteristic such as the reason for shunt placement and age when the shunt was placed. Infection remains a common cause of shunt revisions.

FACTOID

In children studied between 6 and 60 months of age, isoflurane, sevoflurane, and desflurane decreased mean arterial pressure (MAP) and increased intracranial pressure compared to baseline at 0.5 and 1.0 MAC. This resulted in a decrease in cerebral perfusion pressure (CPP). In this study, the effect of MAP on CPP is 3-4 times higher than the effect of the increases in ICP on CPP, making MAP the most important factor in preserving CPP.

36 STATUS EPILEPTICUS

William S. Schechter, MD, MS

YOUR PATIENT

A 5-year-old child is brought to the emergency room for treatment of a tonic-clonic seizure.

The child had been complaining of a "headache" for the past several days and was "out of sorts," according to the mother. The mother administered acetaminophen for a "tactile fever." This morning the child was found unresponsive and hyperextended, having tonic-clonic movements of the extremities while in bed.

Emergency services were called, and after two failed attempts at intubation, Diastat (rectal diazepam) was administered and the child was brought to the emergency department (ED) with a partial nonrebreathing mask in place. On arrival, the child was fitting and cyanotic appearing, and had pinkish foamy secretions about the oropharynx. The child's breathing was stridulous. The eyes were deviated toward the right. Vital signs were HR = 168; BP = 130/90; RR = labored, <8; T = 38.8; SpO_2 = 82%.

PREOPERATIVE CONSIDERATIONS

The first consideration in this case is attainment and maintenance of an adequate airway, oxygenation, and ventilation. Suctioning of the airway, proper placement of a mask, and institution of positive pressure ventilation is foremost. A brief medical history (underlying conditions, trauma, recent infections, metabolic disorders, allergies, and medications) can be elicited by other members of the emergency department team while the airway and intravenous access are being established. Medical attempts at stopping the seizure may be attempted by administering intranasal midazolam (0.2 mg/kg to a maximum of 10 mg) or rectal diazepam (0.2-0.5 mg/kg given only once) until intravenous access is obtained. Given the history, it is likely that the patient is in status epilepticus (seizures lasting more than 30 minutes or recurring episodes of seizure activity without regaining consciousness). It is critical that the seizure be terminated as rapidly as possible to decrease cerebral metabolic stress and hypoxemia. The physical examination is suggestive of an underlying focus.

ANESTHETIC MANAGEMENT

- Support the airway, provide mask ventilation with 100% oxygen, suction oropharynx; rapidly assess airway for ease of intubation. Talk to emergency medical technicians about why they feel previous attempts failed.
- Once IV access is obtained, administer lorazepam, 0.1 mg/kg; this may be repeated if the seizure is not terminated within 5 minutes.
- If the seizure terminates, load with either fosphenytoin in normal saline (10-20 phenytoin equivalent units) or phenobarbital 10-20 mg/kg pending further evaluation.
- If seizure does not terminate promptly, positive pressure ventilation is not assured, or there is evidence of regurgitation, unrelieved upper airway obstruction or pulmonary edema fluid, intubate the trachea.
- It should be noted that local anesthetic–induced seizures occasionally seen after an errant block are a unique subset of status epilepticus; they require immediate intubation and correction of the associated respiratory and metabolic acidosis to prevent local anesthetic toxicity associated with uptake and trapping of the agent intracellularly. Although initially recommended for cardiovascular toxicity, Intralipid 20% may be therapeutic for central nervous system toxicity as well.
- Equipment needed: working laryngoscope handles, appropriate blades, induction agent, relaxants, appropriate airways and endotracheal tubes, suction; have laryngeal mask airway available for a failed intubation/ventilation scenario.
- Identify assistants in the ED and assign their respective roles as part of a resource management protocol.
- Administer an intubating dose of propofol (2-3 mg/kg); have a knowledgeable assistant apply cricoid pressure and intubate. Beware of the significant risk of aspiration (this may have already occurred before arrival at the hospital). A short-acting muscle relaxant may be needed to open the mouth and facilitate intubation. Succinylcholine may be used if it is not otherwise contraindicated. Long-acting relaxants (such as rocuronium, dose 0.8-1 mg/kg) may be used with caution, since they will not allow for rapid assessment of seizure termination and may create problems if intubation and ventilation attempts fail. In regions of the world where suggammadex is available, however, they may be excellent appropriate alternatives.
- Send STAT electrolytes (especially sodium, calcium, and magnesium) and glucose.
- Confirm tube placement directly by laryngoscopy and by noting the equal rise and fall of the chest, equality of breath sounds by auscultation, and sustained CO_2 by capnometry or capnography. Breath sounds may be unequal if aspiration has occurred or if the tube is

malpositioned. Place an orogastric tube and suction the stomach after the endotracheal tube (ETT) is secured at the appropriate depth. Suction the ETT. Obtain a STAT chest x-ray as soon as appropriate.

DOs and DON'Ts

✓ Do obtain a history. A history of trauma may indicate a cervical-spine fracture. You would want to know this before manipulating the airway. A period of lethargy and headache may indicate a space-occupying lesion. Hyperventilation (perhaps with cricoid pressure) and a larger dose of induction agent may be appropriate to prevent herniation during the intubation sequence. A history of fever may require prophylaxis for the emergency responders as well as prompt antibiotic coverage. A history of diabetes may indicate hypoglycemia as a cause.

✓ Do listen to the lungs *before* intubation. This will help you interpret breath sounds, diagnose the possibility of aspiration, and assess proper tube position after intubation.

⊗ Don't administer relaxant unless you are reasonably assured that you can intubate or ventilate or that you have a backup plan (additional equipment, other anesthesia personnel, or surgical airway availability). Significant loading doses of an agent or agents will often be required to terminate a seizure.

✓ Do keep in mind that breathing may stop once enough anticonvulsants are administered to terminate the seizure; ventilation will need to be supported.

✓ Do obtain a STAT glucose level. It is not unusual for glucose levels to be depressed after prolonged seizures (or to be a cause of seizures in metabolically deranged patients).

✓ Do correct electrolyte abnormalities:
- Hypocalcemia ($CaCl_2$ 10-30 mg/kg or calcium gluconate 30-60 mg/kg IV)
- Hypomagnesemia (Mg_2SO_4 25 mg/kg IV)
- Hypoglycemia (dextrose 25% 0.5 mg/kg IV followed by maintenance infusion)
- Hyponatremia *cannot* be rapidly corrected without risk of central pontine myelinolysis. However, 3% hypertonic normal saline may be given at doses of 1-2 mL/kg to raise serum sodium by no more than 3-5 mOsm/L if the initial serum sodium was less than 120 mEq/L in an effort to terminate the seizure if anticonvulsants were ineffective. Further correction must be accomplished over a period of days, and fluid management is determined on the basis of etiology (eg, syndrome of inappropriate antidiuretic hormone, cerebral salt wasting syndrome, or hyponatremic dehydration).

✓ Do check pupillary diameter, response, and eye position after intubation. Hyperventilation may be required transiently if there is a significant bleed or other mass-occupying lesion. This may be indicated by dilated pupils (usually unilateral), in the absence of administration of a muscarinic antagonist, or downward deviation of the eyes.

✓ Do consider the need for further diagnostic testing, such as an emergency CT scan, lumbar puncture complete blood cell count (LP CBC), other chemistries and cultures, and/or empirical antibiotic therapy.

✓ Do confirm that muscle relaxation has dissipated before assuming that seizures have been terminated.

✓ Do empirically load with fosphenytoin or phenobarbital until a diagnosis is established. Nonconvulsive status is part of the differential if consciousness is not regained. An electroencephalogram may be required for diagnosis.

FACTOID

Seizure means to be captured or taken by force, and in less enlightened times implied that an evil spirit or the devil had taken hold of one's body and mind. It is used as a noun. The quaint terminology "fits" or "fitting" is perfectly acceptable nomenclature that may be used to describe a patient who is actively having a seizure and is not to be considered pejorative terminology.

37 CHIARI MALFORMATION

Riva R. Ko, MD

YOUR PATIENT

A 2-year-old girl was recently diagnosed with a Chiari I malformation. The patient has a history of poor feeding and swallowing, as well as decreased sensation in her upper and lower extremities. She presents for posterior fossa decompression.

MRI shows Chiari I malformation without evidence of hydrocephalus.

PREOPERATIVE CONSIDERATIONS

Chiari malformations are structural cerebellar defects in which part of the cerebellum is displaced below the foramen magnum. They are classified by degree of severity and by the parts of the brain that protrude into the spinal canal. In Chiari type I malformations, only the cerebellar tonsils extend into the foramen magnum, without involvement of the brain stem. This is the most common form of Chiari malformation, and it may be asymptomatic until adolescence or even adulthood. Chiari type II malformations (also called Arnold-Chiari malformations) involve extension of both cerebellar and brainstem tissue into the foramen magnum, and are associated with the presence of a myelomeningocele. The rarer Chiari type III and type IV malformations are more serious; type III involves herniation of the cerebellum, brain stem, and possibly the fourth ventricle through the foramen magnum into the spinal canal, while type IV is characterized by cerebellar hypoplasia.

Preoperative evaluation should include a detailed history of any neurologic deficits, as well as any comorbid conditions. There should be extensive discussion with the neurosurgeon prior to the procedure. It is important to know whether or not dural opening is planned, the need for intraoperative neurologic monitoring, the requirement for steroids, and whether or not nonsteroidal anti-inflammatory drugs such as ketorolac will be permissible postoperatively. Parents should be informed that two IV lines and an arterial line will be placed, and that the patient will recover in the pediatric intensive care unit postoperatively with patient-controlled analgesia (PCA) for pain management. A Foley catheter generally is placed only in older patients. A type and crossmatch should be available, although it is rarely necessary to transfuse in these cases. Parents should always be advised that in this or any other neuro-surgical case, there is always a chance that the child will remain intubated postoperatively, although the plan would be to extubate in the operating room (OR). The patient's head will be placed in pins for this procedure, so there is no need for special facial padding when turning the child prone. A nasotracheal intubation may be considered to better ensure stability of the endotracheal tube in the prone position.

Premedication with oral midazolam would not be expected to inter-fere with somatosensory evoked potential (SSEP) monitoring, and should be administered if appropriate. If there are no contraindications, lines can be placed after the patient has been anesthetized with an inhala-tion induction.

Neurophysiologic monitoring, although controversial, is frequently used in Chiari malformation surgery; it consists of monitoring of SSEPs, and possibly brainstem auditory evoked responses (BAERs). This is particularly useful if the surgeons plan to open the dura. In order to facilitate this monitoring, total intravenous anesthesia (TIVA) should be used for the case; this may include infusion of a short-acting narcotic such as remifentanil, a hypnotic such as propofol or midazolam, and possibly a muscle relaxant such as rocuronium or vecuronium. A small amount of a volatile agent is acceptable, but nitrous oxide is best avoided.

ANESTHETIC MANAGEMENT

- Induce the patient on a stretcher, then turn the patient prone onto the OR table after lines are secured and neurophysiologic monitors applied.
- Make sure a stretcher is available throughout the operation in case of an urgent need to turn the patient back to the supine position.
- Use an arterial line plus two IV lines. A Foley catheter is used only in older patients.
- Consider a nasotracheal intubation for greater stability in the prone position.
- If neurophysiologic monitoring is planned, use the TIVA technique with or without a small amount of volatile anesthetic. Remifentanil (0.05-0.5 µg/kg/min) in conjunction with either propofol (100-200 µg/kg/min) or midazolam (0.1 mg/kg/h) infusion works well.
- Muscle relaxants are fine, and may actually enhance SSEP signals; however, at least one twitch should be maintained. Nitrous oxide should be avoided.
- Make sure to deepen the patient prior to placement of the patient's head in pins, especially as this may occur after a long period of rela-tively little stimulation (placement of lines and monitors).

- Use extreme care when positioning the patient prone. In addition to the usual considerations for prone positioning, the surgeon will need to flex the neck a good deal—watch airway pressures closely! Ensure that you can fit a finger between the chin and the chest. If neurophysiologic monitoring is used, make sure that there are no changes in SSEPs after prone positioning.
- After neurophysiologic monitoring is discontinued, turn off infusions and switch to a volatile agent to enable faster wake-up. Titrate in a longer-acting narcotic, such as morphine (0.05-0.1 mg/kg) or hydromorphone (0.01-0.02 mg/kg).

POSTOPERATIVE CONSIDERATIONS

Patients are admitted to the ICU for close observation of neurologic status and for pain control. Pain control usually is accomplished with narcotic PCA, supplemented by ketorolac if the surgeons are amenable. In this young patient, PCA will have to be administered via continuous infusion and clinician boluses as needed (see Chapter 89).

DOs and DON'Ts

✓ Do pay close attention to airway pressures and neurophysiologic monitoring (if used) when positioning the patient prone.

✓ Do have a stretcher immediately available at all times in case the patient needs to be turned supine emergently.

⊗ Avoid nitrous oxide and high doses of volatile agents, as well as frequent large boluses of IV agents.

✓ Do use TIVA, with or without a small amount of volatile agent. Muscle relaxation is useful.

✓ Do ask the surgeon whether or not steroids should be given intraoperatively.

✓ Do titrate long-acting narcotics after discontinuation of neurophysiologic monitoring, and plan for postoperative PCA. Ask the surgeon if ketorolac will be an acceptable adjuvant for postoperative pain.

CONTROVERSIES

- There is evidence to suggest that bony decompression alone, rather than dural opening, may be sufficient in the operative treatment of children with Chiari I malformations. Such an approach is less invasive and theoretically would reduce the risk of potential complications from surgery (see later discussion); however, more research is needed to conclusively support this approach.

- Although neurophysiologic monitoring (eg, SSEP or BAER) is used fairly routinely in surgical decompression of Chiari I malformations, there is not a great deal of evidence to support its utility, especially given the low incidence of perioperative complications.

SURGICAL CONCERNS

Surgical complications are uncommon and are usually associated with dural opening (cerebrospinal fluid leaks, pseudomeningocele). Other rare complications such as aseptic meningitis, hydrocephalus, and hypoglossal paresis generally are associated with intradural manipulation.

FACTOID

Chiari malformations are so named in honor of the Austrian pathologist Hans Chiari, who first described the disease in the late nineteenth century. Although the pathologist Julius Arnold described only one case in an infant with spina bifida, Chiari type II malformations are often referred to as "Arnold-Chiari malformations."

38 MUSCULAR DYSTROPHY

Riva R. Ko, MD

YOUR PATIENT

A 12-year-old boy with a history of Duchenne muscular dystrophy presents for scoliosis surgery. He is wheelchair-bound and uses biphasic positive airway pressure (BiPAP) at night. An echocardiogram performed 3 months ago showed an ejection fraction of 45%. Pulmonary function tests showed a vital capacity 45% of the predicted value.

PREOPERATIVE CONSIDERATIONS

Duchenne muscular dystrophy (DMD), or pseudohypertrophic muscular dystrophy, is the most common muscular dystrophy seen in children. DMD is an X-linked recessive disease associated with a lack of dystrophin. The absence of dystrophin results in instability and increased permeability of the sarcolemma and elevated intracellular calcium. If the sarcolemma is exposed to volatile agents or succinylcholine, this instability and permeability may worsen, leading to a compensatory hypermetabolic response, including hyperkalemia, hyperthermia, tachycardia, and rhabdomyolysis. Beginning in early childhood, DMD is characterized by progressive deterioration of skeletal, cardiac, and smooth muscles. Proximal muscles are affected first, whereas distal muscles, especially calf muscles, may appear hypertrophied. The Gower sign, in which patients use their arms in order to stand up, reflects the severe proximal weakness. Patients frequently are wheelchair-bound by early adolescence. The major causes of morbidity and mortality are respiratory and cardiac failure.

Preoperative evaluation should include pulmonary function testing, if possible. Vital capacity (VC) less than 50% predicted may be associated with the need for postoperative mechanical ventilation, and a VC less than 30% predicted may lead to serious postoperative complications, even with mechanical ventilation. The preoperative oxygen saturation on room air should be noted. Patients with DMD are at increased risk for pneumonia due to their diminished ability to cough and clear secretions. They may be at increased risk of aspiration due to gastrointestinal hypomotility in conjunction with weak laryngeal reflexes. Preoperative electrocardiogram changes may include tall R waves in V_1, deep Q waves in the limb leads, decreased PR intervals, and sinus tachycardia. Mitral regurgitation or mitral valve prolapse may be present as a result of papillary muscle dysfunction. Dilated cardiomyopathy is common in older adolescent patients and is a major cause of mortality.

ANESTHETIC MANAGEMENT

- Flush the anesthesia machine preoperatively (usually 10 L/min for 20 minutes; consult manufacturer) and change the soda lime ("trigger-free technique").
- Avoid succinylcholine and volatile agents. Trigger-free anesthetic (eg, total intravenous anesthesia or regional) is preferred.
- Use an arterial line for measurement of arterial blood gases, electrolytes, and hematocrit.
- Monitor central venous pressure to assess intravascular volume and monitor for congestive heart failure (CHF).
- Prepare to treat acute rhabdomyolysis or hyperkalemia with sodium bicarbonate, insulin, calcium chloride, and mannitol.
- Decompress the stomach with a nasogastric tube.
- Transfuse as necessary to maximize oxygen delivery.
- Monitor urine output closely to assess volume status.
- Use cautious narcotic administration for pain.
- There must be careful attention to positioning the patient, to prevent nerve injuries and to minimize respiratory compromise.

POSTOPERATIVE CONSIDERATIONS

Patients are admitted to the intensive care unit for close observation of respiratory and cardiac status, and for possible postoperative mechanical ventilation. Even if extubated, patients will usually need noninvasive positive pressure ventilation (NPPV) in the postoperative period (patients such as this one, who use BiPAP preoperatively, should certainly be placed on BiPAP postoperatively if they are extubated). DMD patients can have compromised pulmonary function postoperatively due to atelectasis, hypoventilation, and airway secretions. Patients are at risk of congestive heart failure, particularly after major surgery with significant blood loss and/or fluid shifts. Rhabdomyolysis and/or cardiac arrest can occur in DMD patients anywhere from shortly after induction of anesthesia to 20 minutes after arriving in recovery; therefore, vigilance for elevated temperatures, tachycardia, and myoglobinuria must be maintained in seemingly stable patients postoperatively.

DOs and DON'Ts

✓ Do properly flush the anesthesia machine preoperatively and consider the use of a trigger-free technique.

⊗ Do *not* use succinylcholine; strongly consider avoiding volatile agents.

✓ Do have emergency medications available to treat hyperkalemia and/or rhabdomyolysis, eg, sodium bicarbonate, insulin, calcium chloride, and mannitol.

✓ Do decompress the stomach thoroughly with a nasogastric tube.

⊗ Do not allow the patient to become hypovolemic, but be aware of the potential for CHF.

✓ Do have NPPV (eg, BiPAP) available if extubation is planned.

CONTROVERSIES

- It is unclear whether the potential hyperkalemia and rhabdomyolysis associated with DMD truly fall within the MH spectrum; therefore, volatile anesthetic agents are not contraindicated per se, but probably are best avoided if possible. Because of this controversy, it is also uncertain whether or not dantrolene plays a useful role in treating these episodes.
- There is evidence from randomized controlled studies that glucocorticoid corticosteroid therapy in Duchenne muscular dystrophy improves muscle strength and function in the short term (6 months to 2 years), but also causes adverse side effects. Nonrandomized studies show similar outcomes with long-term corticosteroid use.

SURGICAL CONCERNS

Spinal surgery usually is undertaken in an attempt to alleviate the restrictive pulmonary disease caused by progressive kyphoscoliosis. Some surgeons perform spinal surgery in all patients with DMD with even a mild scoliosis (Cobb angle ≤30°) soon after ambulation is lost; this allows for a technically easier surgery in patients who usually do not yet have severe respiratory problems. Patients with onset of scoliosis at under 14 years and a maximal annual deterioration in Cobb angle greater than 20° almost always require surgery. However, other patients may be successfully managed conservatively, so an individualized approach may be warranted. The risk of this more individualized approach, however, is that scoliosis might develop and progress rapidly when the cardiorespiratory function has deteriorated to such a degree that the risks of surgery outweigh the benefits.

FACTOID

Unexplained cardiac arrest and death in children who were subsequently found to have DMD was one of the driving forces behind the issuing of the "black box warning" against the routine use of succinylcholine in children.

39 MYOTONIC DYSTROPHY

Riva R. Ko, MD

YOUR PATIENT

A 13-year-old girl with a history of myotonic dystrophy presents for cholecystectomy for gallstones. She has dysphagia and gastroesophageal reflux disease, and a history of dysrhythmia for which she takes procainamide.

The physical examination showed bilateral ptosis, facial weakness, and markedly decreased strength in distal extremities.

PREOPERATIVE CONSIDERATIONS

Myotonic dystrophy, also known as Steinert's disease, is an autosomal dominant neuromuscular disorder characterized by sustained skeletal muscle contractions in response to stimulation. This is thought to be caused by abnormal chloride conductance in the muscle membrane, and by decreased inactivation of sodium channels. Myotonic episodes can be triggered by pain, stress, cold, and shivering. Myotonic dystrophy occurs in roughly 5 per 100 000 births and can be congenital (the most severe form), early-onset juvenile (usually in the second decade of life), adult-onset, or late-onset asymptomatic. Neonates with congenital myotonic dystrophy frequently present with hypotonia, difficulty feeding, and respiratory distress, and have an associated high mortality; the physical examination typically shows facial weakness, a tent-shaped mouth, and talipes equinovarus. Patients with juvenile myotonic dystrophy may exhibit delayed motor and speech milestones, but signs and symptoms of true muscular degeneration and weakness may not become apparent until after the age of 10. Myotonic dystrophy tends to involve multiple organ systems; common symptoms include cataracts, developmental delay, cardiac conduction abnormalities, aspiration pneumonia, insulin resistance, and thyroid problems.

Preoperative evaluation should include a detailed history of any neurologic deficits, as well as any comorbid conditions. A history of dysphagia and/or frequent aspiration may predict postoperative respiratory complications, and a chest x-ray may be warranted in this setting. At a minimum, this patient should have a baseline electrocardiogram, and a preoperative echocardiogram and/or cardiology consultation may be helpful.

Patients with myotonic dystrophy often have cognitive impairment and may display fear and anxiety preoperatively, which may in itself trigger a myotonic episode. However, patients are very sensitive to the respiratory depressant effects of drugs such as benzodiazepines and opiates. Therefore, premedication with an anxiolytic such as midazolam is controversial, and the risks and benefits must be weighed by the anesthesiologist. Premedication with an antacid is reasonable, particularly in patients with a history of aspiration.

This patient is taking procainamide, which increases the duration of action of muscle relaxants and antagonizes the effects of neostigmine. Procainamide also can potentiate the risk of ventricular arrhythmias in the setting of antihistamines and beta blockers.

ANESTHETIC MANAGEMENT

- Place external pacer/defibrillator pads prior to the induction of anesthesia.
- Consider placement of an arterial line for assessment of adequate oxygenation and ventilation.
- Consider rapid-sequence induction, especially if there is a history of aspiration; however, succinylcholine should be avoided, both because of the possibility of masseter spasm and/or a myotonic episode and because of a possible exaggerated hyperkalemic response due to dystrophic muscle changes. Use IV fluids that do not contain potassium for this reason as well.
- Use a lower dose of hypnotic agent for induction because of the exaggerated apneic response of patients with myotonic dystrophy to these agents.
- Use gentle direct laryngoscopy and jaw manipulation, as patients with myotonic dystrophy are prone to temporomandibular joint dislocation.
- Maintenance of anesthesia can be achieved with either volatile or intravenous agents; however, use of volatile agents may be limited by their myocardial and respiratory depressant effects, while response to IV agents such as propofol is extremely variable and may be associated with awareness.
- Use aggressive measures to keep patients warm, as hypothermia can trigger a myotonic episode: warm the operating room, warm IV fluids, use a forced-air warming blanket, and place a humidifier on the circuit.
- Avoid muscle relaxants, if possible; however, if muscle relaxants are used, shorter-acting agents and lower doses should be chosen. Use of reversal is controversial (see later discussion).
- Use caution with peripheral nerve stimulators; the electrical stimulus in itself could trigger a myotonic episode, which may then be mistaken for sustained tetanus and full reversal of neuromuscular blockade.

- Opioids should be avoided, if possible, as patients with myotonic dystrophy are exquisitely sensitive to their respiratory depressant effects.
- Patients should be extubated only if they meet strict extubation criteria, especially if they have received opioids and/or muscle relaxants.

POSTOPERATIVE CONSIDERATIONS

Patients with myotonic dystrophy are at risk for delayed-onset apnea postoperatively; therefore strong consideration should be given to admitting all patients with myotonic dystrophy to the intensive care unit (ICU) for at least 24 hours for close observation of respiratory status. This is particularly true in patients with a history of respiratory compromise, those undergoing abdominal or thoracic surgery, and those requiring intraoperative or postoperative opioids for pain control. When feasible, use of acetaminophen, nonsteroidal anti-inflammatory drugs (NSAIDs), and/or regional anesthesia is preferable to use of opioids in these patients. Often, it is difficult to ascertain whether or not there are residual anesthetic effects, so if these patients are extubated, equipment and personnel should be available for immediate reintubation if necessary.

DOs and DON'Ts

✓ Do take a careful history, with particular focus on neurologic, cardiac, and gastrointestinal dysfunction.

✓ Do place pacer/defibrillator pads on the patient prior to induction.

✓ Do strongly consider a rapid-sequence induction of anesthesia.

⊗ Do not use succinylcholine. If possible, avoid muscle relaxants altogether.

⊗ Do not use opioids, if possible.

⊗ Do not allow the patient to become cold.

⊗ Do not extubate unless these patients meet strict extubation criteria.

✓ Do strongly consider ICU admission postoperatively for at least 24 hours.

✓ Do consider NSAIDs, acetaminophen, and/or regional anesthesia for postoperative pain.

CONTROVERSIES

Use of neostigmine to reverse neuromuscular blockade in patients with myotonic dystrophy is controversial. There are case reports of myotonic episodes being triggered by the neostigmine itself; however, a recent study about perioperative adverse effects in children with myotonic dystrophy showed a significantly higher risk of pulmonary complications in myotonic patients who received nondepolarizing muscle relaxants but no reversal.

SURGICAL CONCERNS

Sustained myotonic contractions may not be alleviated by administration of muscle relaxants, so surgeons need to be aware that increased muscle tone intraoperatively most likely is not being caused by inadequate muscle relaxation—surgical stimulation and/or use of the Bovie are more likely causes. Surgeons also need to be aware of the need for the operating room to be kept warm at all times so as not to precipitate a myotonic episode.

FACTOID

Myotonic dystrophy exhibits "anticipation," or a tendency to become progressively more severe with successive generations. This seems to be particularly true when the disease is inherited maternally.

40 SPINAL MUSCULAR ATROPHY

William S. Schechter, MD, MS

YOUR PATIENT

A 4-year-old male with spinal muscular atrophy (SMA) presents for vertical expandable prosthetic titanium rib (VEPTR) insertion. He was diagnosed with SMA at 8 months of age. He has gastroesophageal reflux and is fed via a gastrojejunostomy tube. He is wheelchair bound and is dependent on biphasic positive airway pressure (BiPAP). He has reactive airways and is on fluticasone and albuterol.

The physical examination shows a smiling child with obvious scoliosis sitting in a wheelchair. He is verbally communicative but speaks softly in a whispered voice. Venous access is poor.

PREOPERATIVE CONSIDERATIONS

Spinal muscular atrophy is an autosomal recessive disorder that is associated with the death of anterior spinal horn motor neurons. There are several forms of the disease:

Type 1 SMA is a severe form of the disease that manifests during early infancy. Without significant respiratory support, these children will rarely survive beyond infancy or childhood. The most severe form of this disease is often called SMA0. Children with SMA0 rarely survive to adolescence; those with mild forms of SMA1 who receive contemporary excellent, aggressive care, have survived to adulthood.

Type 2 SMA disease patients are moderately affected; presentation is between 6 and 18 months of age. Many children survive to adulthood.

Type 3 SMA patients have a near normal life expectancy.

Type 4 SMA or adult-onset disease manifests in the third decade of life with increasing proximal muscular weakness but near normal life expectancy.

Signs and symptoms can include floppiness early in infancy in the most severely affected; weakness of the appendicular and axial musculature, resulting in a weak cough and cry; poor feeding; failure to thrive; delay in the development of motor milestones; respiratory distress; aspiration pneumonias; areflexia and fasciculations (especially of the tongue). These patients may require noninvasive forms of ventilation such as continuous positive airway pressure, BiPAP, and cough assist devices; in some cases, tracheostomy is required for ventilation or pulmonary toilet. In addition, because of bulbar involvement, feeding may be best accomplished by a gastrostomy tube or gastrojejunostomy. Some children require a fundoplication to prevent aspiration of gastric contents. The development of kyphoscoliosis often requires surgical intervention in the form of fusion or spinal instrumentation to allow patients to sit comfortably and avoid progression of their restrictive pulmonary disease. These patients may have abnormalities of fatty acid oxidation and tend to develop metabolic acidosis during prolonged fasts. Arrhythmias, congenital structural cardiac disease, and decreased myocardial function have been reported in these patients.

VEPTR is a telescoping rod that is applied to the concave side of the deformity; it is designed to prevent the progression of thoracic insufficiency syndrome and theoretically allows for normal chest and consequent lung growth. Unlike spinal fusion and instrumentation, these devices can be expanded intermittently to allow for growth, and the application procedure itself is less invasive and has less potential for catastrophic hemodynamic instability because of blood and fluid loss.

ANESTHETIC MANAGEMENT

- There is a potential risk of aspiration.
- IV placement may be achieved with premedication with midazolam 0.5 mg/kg to a maximum of 20 mg, ELA-Max, or EMLA cream and 50% nitrous oxide in oxygen followed by an IV induction; alternatively, an inhalational induction may be considered. The gastrostomy tube should be vented prior to induction.
- A urinary catheter and two IV lines are needed.
- An arterial line should be placed, an initial hematocrit and blood gas should be taken, and a specimen for a "type and save" should be sent to the blood bank.
- Induction may be carried out utilizing sevoflurane in oxygen with or without nitrous oxide, or intravenous agents such as propofol supplemented by an opioid may be chosen.
- Intubation of the trachea may be performed with or without muscle relaxation. Maintenance of anesthesia may be conducted with a combination of propofol by continuous infusion and an opioid (fentanyl or remifentanil infusion) or by utilizing intermittent dosing of morphine, hydromorphone, or fentanyl. Early extubation of the trachea and institution of BiPAP is preferred except in the most marginal patients or for patients who have had lengthy procedures or significant blood loss or fluid administration.
- Difficult intubation may be associated with atrophy and contractures of the muscles of mastication.

- Significant restrictive disease may be associated with right heart failure; consider an electrocardiogram or echocardiogram.
- The patient is likely to need pediatric intensive care unit care for postoperative pulmonary toilet and early pain management.
- There is a possible need for mechanical ventilation postoperatively. Noninvasive ventilation is likely to be necessary if forced vital capacity (FVC) <50% predicted; FVC <30% predicted suggests a further increase in that risk.
- Consider preoperative training, optimization of medication regimen, and postoperative manual and mechanical cough assist.
- Plan to extubate patients directly to noninvasive positive pressure ventilation, especially if FVC <30%.
- The subsequent lengthening of the VEPTR is a relatively short procedure that typically does not require an arterial line or second IV and can be performed on an outpatient basis in selected patients after a period of postanesthesia observation.

DOs and DON'Ts

✓ Do take meticulous care of pulmonary toilet (suction carefully, maintain airway humidification, and use cough assist before starting the case).
✓ Do position carefully and keep warm; there are increased radiative losses due to a higher body surface area (BSA)/weight ratio.
✓ Monitor for pneumothorax or hemothorax.
⊗ Don't commit to postoperative ventilation early in the case.
✓ Do maintain a slightly head-up position when prone; consider early colloid use for blood loss replacement, and make certain that there is no pressure on the eyes in an effort to prevent postoperative amaurosis.
⊗ Don't give succinylcholine to avoid the risk of severe hyperkalemia (no additional risk for malignant hyperthermia).

CONTROVERSIES

Preoperative arterial blood gases and pulmonary function testing may be helpful, but are often unavailable; preoperative discussion with the pulmonologist is often most helpful.

FACTOID

Orthopedics means *straight child*. Since its inception as a medical specialty, it has been concerned with the correction of congenital musculoskeletal anomalies and *straightening of the child*.

41 SELECTIVE DORSAL RHIZOTOMY

Riva R. Ko, MD

YOUR PATIENT

A 4-year-old girl with a history of cerebral palsy and severe spasticity presents for selective dorsal rhizotomy (SDR). She is taking baclofen and tizanidine. History and physical examination are otherwise unremarkable.

PREOPERATIVE CONSIDERATIONS

Spasticity in children usually is caused by cerebral palsy (CP), traumatic brain injury, or spinal cord injury, and can lead to a significantly decreased quality of life. Nonsurgical treatment consists of physical and occupational therapy and oral spasmolytic drugs; invasive options include injections of botulinum toxin, localized orthopedic procedures, intrathecal baclofen (ITB) pump implantation, and SDR. In spastic CP, there is increased alpha motor neuron activity and spasticity due to cerebral hemispheric damage. The goal of SDR is to decrease the excitation of these alpha motor neurons and thus alleviate spasticity, while preserving motor and sensory function. Unlike ITB, SDR mainly improves spasticity of the lower extremities; it does not significantly improve dystonia. SDR usually involves electrophysiologically guided severing of dorsal rootlets from L2 to S1 or S2. The decision as to which dorsal rootlets to cut can be based on the motor responses to stimulation, clinical history, or a combination of the two.

Many children presenting for SDR will have a history of prematurity and associated neonatal lung disease, so there may be intra- or postoperative respiratory complications. Intravenous access and positioning may be difficult because of spasticity. The patient will need to be placed in the prone position for surgery, with all the attendant potential complications.

Antispasticity drugs such as baclofen should not be discontinued preoperatively, as this may precipitate acute withdrawal.

ANESTHETIC MANAGEMENT

- Carefully position patients prone with appropriate padding.
- Avoid muscle relaxants to allow for intraoperative electrical stimulation and electromyogram (a one-time dose of muscle relaxant for intubation is acceptable).

- Although children with spastic CP are not at increased risk of succinylcholine-induced hyperkalemia, there may be associated increased muscle spasm and rigidity, so succinylcholine is best avoided.
- Volatile anesthetics are a good choice for maintenance of anesthesia, since they do not interfere with electrophysiologic monitoring in SDR. Intraoperative supplementation with narcotics may be useful.
- Dorsal rootlet stimulation may cause bradycardia and/or hypotension; this may be transient and self-limited, but it may require treatment with atropine.
- Avoid aggressive measures to warm patients undergoing SDR, as there may be increased metabolic heat production from stimulation of the lower extremities.
- Avoid ketamine, as it may alter the response to electrical stimulation.

POSTOPERATIVE CONSIDERATIONS

Although patients can usually be extubated at the end of SDR, they require intensive care unit observation, primarily for management of postoperative pain. Patients experience significant pain after SDR, due to both multilevel laminectomies and manipulation of nerve roots. Patients generally require continuous narcotic infusions, supplemented by nonsteroidal anti-inflammatory drugs and benzodiazepines. Postoperative fever is common, and is thought to be caused by atelectasis or chemical meningitis.

DOs and DON'Ts

✓ Do position patients carefully in the prone position using appropriate padding.
✓ Do use volatile agents for induction and/or maintenance of anesthesia.
✓ Do supplement with intraoperative narcotics as needed.
⊗ Do not use muscle relaxants during the case.
⊗ Do not use succinylcholine at all, if possible.
⊗ Do not aggressively warm patients.
✓ Do be prepared to treat possible bradycardia and hypotension associated with dorsal rootlet stimulation.
✓ Do aggressively treat any postoperative pain.
⊗ Do not allow the patient to become too warm or too cold.

CONTROVERSIES

- While most institutions employ a surgical technique involving electrophysiologic guidance of dorsal rootlet severing, there is some evidence to support good outcomes using a surgical technique based on clinical history alone.

SURGICAL CONCERNS

Given the many therapeutic options available to treat spastic CP, if and when to undertake a permanent, invasive measure such as SDR is controversial. However, the longstanding history of SDR's efficacy and safety when performed in the appropriate patient population (see later discussion) makes it an appealing option to many parents.

FACTOID

A study in the United Kingdom demonstrated the surprising result of significant weight gain after SDR, perhaps reflecting an improvement in spasticity, which itself consumes energy.

42 MYASTHENIA GRAVIS

Riva R. Ko, MD

YOUR PATIENT

An 11-year-old girl with myasthenia gravis presents for thymectomy. The patient has a history of ptosis, dysphagia, and generalized muscle weakness.

The medications she is using are pyridostigmine and prednisone.

PREOPERATIVE CONSIDERATIONS

Myasthenia gravis (MG) is an autoimmune disease in which antibodies are directed against the acetylcholine receptor at the neuromuscular junction. The disease is characterized by weakness and easy fatigability of voluntary muscles. Common symptoms include ptosis, diplopia, dysphagia, and dysarthria. Weakness of respiratory muscles may be severe during a myasthenic crisis. There are three types of myasthenia gravis that present in the pediatric population. Neonatal MG is a transient disorder caused by the passage of antibodies across the placenta from mothers who have MG, which may occur in 20%-30% of infants born to affected mothers. Congenital myasthenia is an autosomal recessive condition affecting the motor endplate. Juvenile MG usually presents in children over the age of 10, has a female predominance, and tends to have a presentation similar to that of the MG seen in adults: autoimmune in nature, often associated with an abnormal thymus gland, and classified as affecting either ocular muscles only or all voluntary muscles. Symptoms of MG worsen with exercise and tend to improve with rest. Medical therapy consists of treatment with cholinesterase inhibitors such as pyridostigmine and neostigmine to increase the available level of acetylcholine at the neuromuscular junction, as well as steroids to suppress the immune response. In a myasthenic crisis, IV immunoglobulin (IVIG) and/or plasmapheresis may be necessary. Surgical treatment with thymectomy can be curative, as antibodies to the acetylcholine receptor are produced by the thymus. Because of potential immunosuppression, thymectomy usually is deferred until the patient is at least 10 years old.

Preoperative evaluation should include a detailed history of the severity of weakness, specifically regarding bulbar and respiratory muscles. Pulmonary function tests are helpful if the child is cooperative.

Anticholinesterase medications increase airway secretions, potentiate narcotic effects, increase sensitivity to nondepolarizing muscle relaxants, and inhibit the metabolism of succinylcholine and ester local anesthetics. Ideally, anticholinesterase medications would be discontinued preoperatively, and the patient would be scheduled as the first case. However, discontinuation of anticholinesterase therapy in children with severe MG may cause aspiration or respiratory failure, so in these patients, medications are continued until surgery. Because of the autoimmune nature of MG, there is an association with thyroid dysfunction, which should be evaluated during the preoperative assessment.

Sedative premedication should be avoided because of possible potentiation effects of anticholinesterase therapy. Consider premedication with an anticholinergic drug such as glycopyrrolate to decrease excess salivation.

ANESTHETIC MANAGEMENT

- Continue any preoperative corticosteroids, and supplement with intraoperative stress dose hydrocortisone.
- Induction and maintenance can be done with either volatile agents or IV agents such as propofol and remifentanil.
- Do invasive blood pressure monitoring for the surgery itself, as well as for postoperative arterial blood gases.
- Avoid hypothermia and hypokalemia, which may worsen marginal respiratory function.
- Avoid drugs that may precipitate a myasthenic crisis, such as anticonvulsants and aminoglycosides.
- Patients with MG may require 2-4 times the normal dose of succinylcholine to achieve a depolarizing block; however, phase II block may occur, and anticholinesterase therapy may inhibit the breakdown of succinylcholine, so it should be avoided if possible.
- Avoid nondepolarizing muscle relaxants (NDMRs) if possible; if they must be given, use greatly decreased doses.
- Monitor neuromuscular blockade at the facial nerve, since this may overestimate neuromuscular blockade in patients with ocular weakness.
- Patients taking perioperative anticholinesterase therapy may exhibit a decreased response to the anticholinesterase reversal of NDMRs; reversal can also precipitate a cholinergic crisis, which is difficult to differentiate from a myasthenic crisis. IV edrophonium can be administered to differentiate between the two.
- Extubation should be attempted as early as possible if bulbar and respiratory function appear to be adequate. Be prepared for possible reintubation.

POSTOPERATIVE CONSIDERATIONS

Patients are admitted to the intensive care unit for close observation of respiratory status and titration of postoperative anticholinesterase medications. Opioids must be titrated carefully, and should be supplemented with nonsteroidal anti-inflammatory drugs if surgically permissible. Cholinergic crisis is rare after thymectomy; however, persistent weakness after thymectomy may necessitate IV neostigmine 0.01-0.04 mg/kg IM/IV/SQ with anticholinergic or IVIG therapy. Care should be taken to avoid infection, fever, or stress, which may precipitate a myasthenic crisis.

DOs and DON'Ts

✓ Do continue corticosteroids preoperatively and intraoperatively.
⊗ If possible, do not use succinylcholine.
✓ Do consider using remifentanil and propofol for maintenance of anesthesia.
⊗ If possible, do not use nondepolarizing muscle relaxants.
✓ Do attempt extubation as early as respiratory status permits.
⊗ Do not give patients with MG anticonvulsant or aminoglycoside drugs, as these can precipitate a myasthenic crisis.

CONTROVERSIES

- There is debate as to the optimal timing of thymectomy for juvenile MG. Fear of autoimmune problems has prompted many surgeons to defer performing thymectomy until the onset of puberty; however, this has not been borne out in the limited available studies. There also is greater chance of spontaneous remission in children with earlier onset of MG. There is some evidence to suggest that thymectomy should be performed within 2 years after the onset of symptoms to maximize the opportunity for remission.
- It also is uncertain whether certain ethnicities may derive more benefit from thymectomy than others. Most studies show a beneficial effect in white children; there appears to be a beneficial effect in African American children as well, but data are much more limited. There may not be much benefit in Asian patients, since they have both a higher incidence of ocular MG and a higher rate of spontaneous remission.
- A thoracic epidural may help with intra- and postoperative analgesia, but it will have to be combined with general anesthesia because of the need for a very high block.

SURGICAL CONCERNS

Thymectomy usually is performed via a complete sternotomy, an upper sternal split, or a cervical approach. If thoracoscopic thymectomy is performed, one-lung ventilation may be necessary, which can be achieved with a double lumen endotracheal tube, a bronchial blocker, or endobronchial intubation.

FACTOID

Neither neonatal MG nor congenital MG is associated with an abnormal thymus, so thymectomy is not performed for either of these two conditions.

43 MOYAMOYA DISEASE

Riva R. Ko, MD

YOUR PATIENT

A 2-year-old girl recently had an ischemic stroke. Cerebral angiography confirmed the diagnosis of moyamoya disease. She presents for encephaloduroarteriosynangiosis (EDAS).

Laboratory: Thyroid-stimulating hormone 0.25
Physical examination: Right hemiparesis

PREOPERATIVE CONSIDERATIONS

- Moyamoya disease is a rare cause of strokes in children, characterized by progressive stenosis of the distal internal carotid and basilar arteries. Affected children present with ischemic stroke, transient ischemic attacks (TIAs), and headache, and symptoms may be exacerbated by crying or straining; adults may present with intracranial hemorrhage.
- Medical therapy with vasodilators such as calcium channel blockers and antiplatelet drugs such as aspirin does not prevent progression of the disease.
- Surgical intervention aims to increase collateral cerebral blood flow (CBF) via either direct or indirect revascularization. In adults, direct revascularization usually is accomplished with a superficial temporal artery (STA) to middle cerebral artery bypass, but this is technically difficult in children. The most common indirect revascularization surgery in children is EDAS, in which the STA is dissected free and then sutured to the edges of the opened dura.
- A history of frequent TIAs suggests decreased CBF and may predict perioperative complications. Medications should be taken until the day of surgery. Patients should be kept as hydrated as possible within nothing by mouth guidelines to maintain CBF.
- Crying can lead to cerebral ischemia in patients with moyamoya disease, since crying leads to hyperventilation and hypocapnia, which in turn may cause cerebral vasoconstriction and decreased CBF. Therefore, premedication with an anxiolytic such as midazolam is recommended.

ANESTHETIC MANAGEMENT

- Avoid hyperventilation and hypotension with induction (whether inhalational or IV).
- Minimize response to laryngoscopy and intubation with opioids and lidocaine to prevent increases in cerebral oxygen consumption ($CMRO_2$). Avoid ketamine.
- Maintain normocarbia to prevent cerebral vasoconstriction and ischemia.
- Maintain normothermia; hyperthermia causes increased $CMRO_2$ and potential cerebral ischemia, while hypothermia may cause cerebral vasospasm and stroke.
- Maintain BP ≥ baseline: use invasive BP monitoring, aggressive hydration, and pressors as needed.
- Crystalloid solutions should not contain glucose.
- Maintain hematocrit >30% to prevent cerebral ischemia. Monitor urine output closely to assess volume status.

POSTOPERATIVE CONSIDERATIONS

Pain control is critical to prevent increased cerebral metabolism and possible stroke; this usually is accomplished with narcotic patient-controlled analgesia.

DOs and DON'Ts

- ✓ Do premedicate with midazolam to prevent crying and agitation on induction.
- ⊗ Do not hyperventilate the patient during either induction or maintenance of anesthesia.
- ✓ Do use opioids and lidocaine to attenuate the response to laryngoscopy and intubation.
- ✓ Do keep the patient well hydrated and maintain BP ≥ baseline.
- ✓ Do aggressively treat any postoperative pain.
- ⊗ Do not allow the patient to become too warm or too cold.

CONTROVERSIES

- Use of total intravenous anesthesia or inhalation anesthesia.
- Usefulness of cerebral monitoring (eg, transcranial Doppler or nearinfrared spectroscopy).

SURGICAL CONCERNS

Beneficial effects of EDAS are delayed because it takes at least 3-4 months for collaterals to develop, and in the interim, there is a risk of perioperative ischemic stroke.

FACTOID

The word *moyamoya* is Japanese for "puff of smoke," taken from the appearance of abnormal collateral vessels on cerebral angiography.

44 TETHERED SPINAL CORD

E. Heidi Jerome, MD

YOUR PATIENT

An 8-year-old boy has a history of urinary incontinence and progressive sensorimotor deficits of the lower extremities. MRI revealed a tethered spinal cord. He presents for neurosurgical release of his tethered cord.

Physical examination shows a sacral dimple.

PREOPERATIVE CONSIDERATIONS

Patients with VACTERL syndrome (vascular abnormalities, anal atresia, cardiac defects, tracheoesophageal fistula, renal abnormalities, and limb defects) may have a tethered cord. However, most patients with a tethered cord, whether presenting as toddlers or as school-age children, are otherwise healthy.

Although a sacral dimple is often the reason for obtaining a spine MRI, sacral dimples are usually not associated with cord abnormalities. However, lumbar skin lesions such as hair tufts, fatty pads, or dimples are often manifestations of spinal abnormalities such as lipomeningocele or dermal sinus tracts, which may cause a tethered spinal cord.

ANESTHETIC MANAGEMENT

Tethered cord release is performed in the prone position with neural monitoring of lower extremity motor and sensory responses and monitoring of the rectal sphincter innervation. Therefore, the anesthetic induction may take place with the patient supine on a stretcher. After endotracheal intubation, Foley catheter placement, and electrode placement for neuromonitoring, the patient is turned prone. Muscle relaxant may be used prior to endotracheal intubation but should be avoided thereafter to allow motor response testing. The anesthetic should be tailored to allow evoked response recordings by keeping the concentration of potent inhaled agents low and using continuous infusions of propofol and remifentanil.

An arterial line is often placed, particularly if laminectomy will be performed at several levels, although blood transfusion is rarely required even in these cases. Surgery may last for 4-6 hours, particularly in older children. One or two intravenous lines should be placed. A bladder catheter should be placed.

The prone position requires special attention to head, chest, and pelvis support. After the endotracheal tube, orogastric tube, esophageal temperature probe, bladder catheter, and anterior electrodes for evoked potential monitoring are placed, the patient is turned to the prone position. The head may be turned to the side or supported in the midline. The endotracheal tube should remain visible, and the eyes, nose, ears, and mouth should be checked to avoid pressure injury. Support of the upper chest and pelvis can be obtained with 2 bolsters or rolls alongside the trunk or a transverse chest roll and a larger roll under the hips. The abdominal wall should be free to expand without pressure during inspiration, which allows normal ventilator pressures and avoids increased pressure in epidural veins that might increase blood loss. Genitalia must be free from pressure. Arms will be positioned with elbows flexed and hands near the head. Posterior and anal electrodes will be placed prior to draping the patient for surgery.

POSTOPERATIVE CONSIDERATIONS

Following tethered cord release, the patient will need to remain flat for several days to avoid leakage of cerebrospinal fluid through the lumbar dura. This may be more readily accomplished in the pediatric intensive care unit, where the nurses can observe the patient. Neural function of the lower extremities can also be checked readily in the intensive care setting. This patient, who has impaired neurologic function preoperatively due to the tethered cord, may not have full recovery of function.

DOs and DON'Ts

✓   Do induce anesthesia on a separate stretcher.
⊗   Don't use muscle relaxant during surgery.
✓   Do check patient's position carefully after prone positioning.

CONTROVERSIES

Although sacrococcygeal dimples are not often associated with spinal cord pathology, most patients with dimples will have sacral ultrasound or MR imaging of the lumbosacral spine performed.

Evoked responses and sphincter electromyograms are becoming the standard of care during these neurosurgical procedures, even though nerve damage is rare.

SURGICAL CONSIDERATIONS

Because early diagnosis of spinal cord lesions is possible with MRI, many patients with a tethered cord will present for surgery as toddlers. Release of the tethered cord is often done prophylactically.

PART 6

HEMATOLOGY/ONCOLOGY

45 WILMS' TUMOR

Teeda Pinyavat, MD

YOUR PATIENT

An 18-month-old boy presents with abdominal distention and a firm, mobile, nontender mass on the right side. His BP is 140/60. Abdominal CT reveals a right renal mass with no extension to surrounding structures. Chest x-ray (CXR) is clear. Urinalysis is positive for red blood cells. He is treated with captopril and scheduled for a right nephrectomy.

PREOPERATIVE CONSIDERATIONS

Wilms' tumor is the most common childhood abdominal malignancy. While these tumors are usually confined to a single kidney, 5% are bilateral, and a small number of patients have intravascular tumor extension to the inferior vena cava (IVC) and right atrium. About 10% are associated with syndromes such as Beckwith-Wiedemann, Soto's, Denys-Drash, WAGR (Wilms' tumor, aniridia, genitourinary anomalies, and mental retardation), and trisomy 18.

The most common presentation is in an otherwise healthy child with increasing abdominal girth and a palpable mass. Malaise, vomiting, constipation, weight loss, anemia, pain, fever, and hematuria can also occur. Hypertension, possibly due to high renin levels, is present in more than 50% of patients at the time of diagnosis and is usually managed with an angiotensin-converting enzyme inhibitor. Other paraneoplastic phenomena may include acquired von Willebrand's disease and hyperaldosteronism.

Preoperative workup should include imaging assessment of local tumor extension (abdominal CT/MRI, pyelogram, and vena cavogram, and echocardiogram if the tumor extends to the IVC and the right atrium) and workup for metastatic disease (CXR or chest CT). Patients with bilateral disease, unresectable disease, or IVC or atrial extension will undergo chemotherapy and radiation treatment prior to resection. Commonly used chemotherapy drugs and their side effects include actinomycin (hepatic dysfunction, myelosuppression, coagulopathy, gastrointestinal upset, immunosuppression), vincristine (peripheral neuropathy, syndrome of inappropriate antidiuretic hormone), and doxorubicin (arrhythmias and cardiomyopathy). Lab studies needed include complete blood cell count, serum chemistries, coagulation studies, and type and cross. Anemia can result from tumor bleeding or myelosuppression. Hypokalemia can result from vomiting, renal potassium wasting (due to hyperaldosteronism), and polydipsia (due to high renin levels). Renal dysfunction is uncommon. Anemia, thrombocytopenia, and electrolyte abnormalities should be corrected preoperatively, and the patient should be well hydrated.

ANESTHETIC MANAGEMENT

- Because of abdominal distention and delayed gastric emptying, treat patient as having a full stomach. Rapid-sequence induction is usually appropriate if airway assessment is normal.
- Patients with overgrowth syndromes causing macroglossia or trisomy 18 causing micrognathia may require specialized airway equipment for intubation.
- Ventilation may become difficult during the case, as intra-abdominal pressure increases as a result of surgical retraction. Consider the use of a low-pressure cuffed endotracheal tube.
- Hypotension on induction may occur if the patient is not well hydrated. Exaggerated hypertension can also occur with intubation if it is present preoperatively.
- Prepare for large intraoperative blood loss and third space fluid losses. This includes access (two large-bore IVs), monitoring (arterial line and possibly central line), and blood products.
- Muscle relaxant should be used and stomach contents emptied to improve surgical exposure.
- A Foley catheter should be placed to help monitor fluid status.
- Blood pressure lability should be expected due to tumor manipulation, intermittent IVC compression, and hypovolemia. Fluids and phenylephrine are useful for hypotension. Increasing anesthetic depth and short-acting vasodilators such as sodium nitroprusside (starting dose 0.3 µg/kg/min, average dose 3 µg/kg/min), phentolamine (1 mg IV bolus as needed), and esmolol (50-200 µg/kg/min) are useful for hypertension.
- A low thoracic epidural (T9/10) is a good adjunct to general anesthesia for postoperative pain control. Consider loading at the end of the procedure if the tumor is large and intraoperative fluid shifts are likely to cause blood pressure lability.

POSTOPERATIVE CONSIDERATIONS

Postoperative bleeding is a risk, as dissection has occurred around major vessels. Postoperative mechanical ventilation may be needed if the patient received large volumes of fluid/products for resuscitation or if a prolonged procedure leads to atelectasis.

DOs and DON'Ts

✓ Do place IVs above the diaphragm (upper extremities, external jugular) due to the possibility of IVC compression or resection.

⊗ Do not place a central line without imaging. The line may dislodge fragments of tumor or thrombus that are present in the vena cava or right atrium.

✓ Do place an arterial line, as blood pressure can be very labile.

✓ Carefully monitor central temperature and use a forced air blanket and warmed fluids.

✓ Do use short-acting agents such as remifentanil, sodium nitroprusside, and esmolol to treat hypertension intraoperatively.

⊗ Do not use long-acting beta blockers and dexmedetomidine, as they will block the normal tachycardic response to hypotension.

⊗ Do not use nitrous oxide, as this can cause further abdominal distention, decreasing surgical exposure and adequacy of ventilation.

✓ Do be vigilant for signs of pulmonary embolism. Tumor embolism into the heart or pulmonary arteries can occur with manipulation of metastases in the IVC.

✓ Do consider the use of epidural for pain control. However, if the IVC is blocked by tumor, epidural vessels may become engorged, leading to increased risk of epidural hematoma.

CONTROVERSIES

It is controversial whether or not asymptomatic lung metastases seen on chest CT only (and not CXR) should affect staging and treatment of these patients.

SURGICAL CONCERNS

If the tumor is confined to the kidney (stage I), the surgeon must be careful not to disrupt the renal capsule. Rupture of the capsule and spillage of the tumor into the peritoneal cavity results in an increase in staging to II or III and alters subsequent treatment.

FACTOIDS

Wilms' tumor is named after a German surgeon who described a series of seven cases in 1899.

In a small number of patients, the tumor secretes erythropoietin, causing polycythemia.

Hypertension usually corrects within a month after surgical resection.

46 ANTERIOR MEDIASTINAL MASS

Teeda Pinyavat, MD

YOUR PATIENT

A 7-year-old child presents with a 3-week history of shortness of breath and a cough that is worse at night. Chest x-ray reveals a large mass in the chest. He presents for a lymph node biopsy under general anesthesia.

> *Physical examination*: No signs of respiratory distress or pallor with supine position; saturation 98% on room air.
> *Imaging*: CT: Anterior mediastinal mass causing slight tracheal deviation to the right and 20% tracheal compression. Echocardiogram: Normal biventricular function; no evidence of external compression.

PREOPERATIVE CONSIDERATIONS

Anterior mediastinal mass can lead to life-threatening airway compression and impingement on the heart and great vessels, leading to cardiovascular collapse upon induction of anesthesia. Mortality is especially high in children, possibly because of a more pliable rib cage and difficulty in symptomatic assessment preoperatively. The most common causes of anterior mediastinal mass in children are Hodgkin's lymphoma, non-Hodgkin's lymphoma, and acute lymphoblastic leukemia.

Respiratory symptoms include dyspnea, orthopnea, cyanosis, cough, wheezing, and stridor. Acute respiratory failure is rare. Cardiovascular symptoms include syncope, sudden pallor, headache, and facial swelling that is worse with Valsalva, and on physical examination jugular venous distention, facial/neck edema, blood pressure changes with postural changes, and increased pulsus paradoxus.

Even asymptomatic children may have significant airway and cardiovascular compression and require imaging studies. CT scan, echocardiogram, and lung function tests are commonly obtained. Severe airway compression is indicated by a tracheal cross section <50% of predicted, severe narrowing at the level of a mainstem bronchus, or peak expiratory flow <50% of predicted. These patients may warrant further diagnostic procedures under local anesthesia with minimal sedation or empiric treatment with steroids, chemotherapy, and/or radiation prior to a general anesthetic. Childhood lymphomas are extremely sensitive to radiation and steroids and can shrink markedly following short courses of treatment. For this reason, part of the tumor may be shielded from radiation to make it available for further workup.

ANESTHETIC MANAGEMENT

- Determine what position provides symptomatic relief (for example, right lateral decubitus or head of bed elevated) and consider placing patient in that position during induction and possibly for the duration of the procedure.
- Place an IV prior to induction, preferably in a lower extremity.
- If cardiovascular symptoms are present, consider arterial line placement prior to induction.
- Maintain spontaneous ventilation during induction with inhalational agent or IV agents (propofol-remifentanil infusion, dexmedetomidine-remifentanil infusion, or ketamine).
- During induction, slowly take over control of ventilation; continuous positive airway pressure may be helpful.
- If intubating, consider the use of a reinforced endotracheal tube, a smaller-sized tube, and mainstem intubation based on the area of compression.
- Consider avoiding muscle relaxants, as they may decrease chest wall tone and increase the risk of airway compromise.
- Have a rigid bronchoscope and operator (ear, nose, and throat [ENT] surgeon) available in the event of tracheal or bronchial collapse.
- If cardiovascular collapse is a concern, preparation should be made for emergent initiation of cardiopulmonary bypass (prepare groins for femoral cannulation, prime pump, have a cardiothoracic surgeon present and scrubbed) or sternotomy to lift the mass.

POSTOPERATIVE CONSIDERATIONS

Intensive care unit admission is usually necessary. The patient may remain intubated and postoperatively is at risk for respiratory and cardiovascular compromise.

DOs and DON'Ts

✓ Do make a careful preoperative assessment, focusing on pulmonary and cardiac symptoms and their relation to positioning. Look at the CT scan to assess for compression of the trachea, carina, and/or mainstem bronchi as well as compression of great vessels and the heart.

(continued)

⊗   Do not make the patient apneic or paralyze the patient prior to establishing the ability to ventilate using positive pressure.

✓   Do coordinate care with ENT and cardiothoracic surgeons and ensure their immediate availability, as required by your preoperative assessment.

⊗   Do not induce anesthesia in the supine position if the patient is symptomatic.

✓   Do ensure adequate vascular access and consider arterial line placement prior to induction.

CONTROVERSIES

- Utility of lung function tests in preoperative evaluation
- Empiric treatment with steroids and radiation prior to a diagnostic biopsy and its effect on biopsy results
- Use of muscle relaxants

SURGICAL CONCERNS

The surgical team must use a multidisciplinary, stepwise approach to the evaluation of a patient with an anterior mediastinal mass and choose the least invasive method of diagnosis and treatment. Diagnoses can sometimes be made by bone marrow aspiration, pleural fluid aspiration, or punch needle biopsy.

FACTOID

Due to increased awareness of anesthetic risk and better preoperative planning, children with anterior mediastinal mass are more likely to have major airway complications in the postoperative period.

47 OSTEOSARCOMA

Teeda Pinyavat, MD

YOUR PATIENT

A 14-year-old boy presents with right knee pain and swelling. Workup reveals a high-grade osteosarcoma in the right proximal tibia without metastasis. After 10 weeks of treatment with methotrexate, doxorubicin, and cisplatin, he now presents for wide resection of the proximal tibia and knee reconstruction. Laboratory findings are: white blood cells 3; hemoglobin 8; hematocrit 24; platelets 130. Chest x-ray, electrocardiogram, and echocardiogram are normal.

PREOPERATIVE CONSIDERATIONS

A careful history and physical examination are important, and special attention should be paid to preoperative pain level and neurologic exam. In anticipation of blood loss, a type and screen, complete blood cell count, and possibly coagulation studies should be obtained. Preoperative embolization may be considered for highly vascular tumors.

Adjuvant chemotherapy is commonly used to treat patients with osteosarcoma, and each agent's systemic effects must be evaluated. Doxorubicin (Adriamycin) is an anthracycline antibiotic that can lead to myelosuppression (anemia, thrombocytopenia, neutropenia), and cardiomyopathy (arrhythmias, heart failure). Cisplatin is a DNA-altering drug that can lead to myelosuppression, nephrotoxicity, nausea/vomiting, peripheral neuropathy, and syndrome of inappropriate diuretic hormone. Methotrexate is an antimetabolite that can lead to myelosuppression, mucositis, diarrhea, pulmonary toxicity, and neurotoxicity at high doses.

ANESTHETIC MANAGEMENT

- A permanent central line used for chemotherapy may be available for induction. Sterile technique should be applied when accessing the line.
- Tumors are usually very vascular, and blood loss can be significant. Obtain adequate IV access, including either two large peripheral IVs or one IV and a central line. An arterial line should be placed to check serial hematocrits.

- Consider placement of a lumbar epidural or peripheral nerve block for intraoperative and postoperative pain management. Loading an epidural during the case will cause a sympathectomy and may lead to intraoperative hypotension. Typically a minimal platelet count of $100 \times 10^9/L$ is required for neuroaxial techniques.
- Positioning: Ensure padding of the operating room table and all extremities. If the patient is in lateral decubitus position, an axillary roll is necessary to prevent nerve injury and decreased blood flow to the dependent arm. Perfusion to the dependent arm should be monitored periodically. Check dependent eyes and ears for pressure.
- Have blood products available. Cell saver cannot be used because of potential tumor spread.
- Bone cement implantation syndrome may cause acute hypoxia and hypotension around the time of cementing, prosthesis insertion, or tourniquet deflation. Etiologies include a combination of the following: reaction to methyl methacrylate monomers, emboli of medullary bone contents under pressure from cement expansion, histamine release, and complement activation. Treatment is supportive.

POSTOPERATIVE CONSIDERATIONS

Postoperative intubation and intensive care unit monitoring may be necessary for the first 24-48 hours. Possible strategies for pain management (including epidural; peripheral nerve blocks; IV patient-controlled analgesia; and use of adjuvant agents such as ketamine, gabapentin, nonsteroidal anti-inflammatory drugs, and methadone) should be considered.

DOs and DON'Ts

✓ Do carefully assess the medication history, including chemotherapeutic agents, and know their systemic effects.

✓ Do withdraw 5 mL before flushing a central line to remove heparin and potential clots.

✓ Do know that flushing a line that is colonized with bacteria could result in sepsis and hypotension.

✓ Do secure the airway properly and position it carefully, as the case could be long.

✓ Do place a pulse oximeter probe on the dependent arm when the patient is in lateral decubitus position to monitor perfusion.

⊗ Do not abduct arms more than 90 degrees to prevent brachial plexus injury.

✓ Do check platelet count and know the plan for deep vein thrombosis prophylaxis prior to placement of an epidural catheter.

CONTROVERSIES

While the use of antifibrinolytic agents (tranexamic acid and aminocaproic acid) has been shown to reduce perioperative blood loss and transfusion in some types of pediatric surgery (cardiac, scoliosis, craniosynostosis), their use in oncologic patients is controversial because of a potential baseline hypercoagulable state.

SURGICAL CONCERNS

Limb-sparing tumor resection may require major neurovascular dissection, removal of significant amounts of bone and soft tissue, reconstruction of bones and joints, creation of muscle flaps, and skin grafting. Therefore, a lengthy procedure with large fluid shifts and blood loss should be anticipated.

FACTOID

Osteosarcoma is the most common bone malignancy in children. Because it is associated with rapid bone growth, osteosarcoma usually presents in the teenage years (average age 15) in long bones (50% around the knee, also common in upper arm), and is more common in males than in females. In some cases, osteosarcoma is hereditary and has been linked to hereditary retinoblastoma.

48 POSTTRANSPLANT LYMPHOPROLIFERATIVE DISORDER

Teeda Pinyavat, MD

YOUR PATIENT

An 8-year-old male who had an orthotopic heart transplant at age 3 for idiopathic cardiomyopathy presents with noisy breathing, snoring at night, and daytime somnolence. He is found to have markedly enlarged adenoids and tonsils as well as cervical lymphadenopathy. He presents to the operating room for tonsillectomy/adenoidectomy and cervical lymph node biopsy. His last catheterization shows no signs of rejection and normal biventricular function.

PREOPERATIVE CONSIDERATIONS

Posttransplant lymphoproliferative disorder (PTLD) encompasses a wide range of disorders, from benign lymphoid tissue hyperplasia (lymph nodes, tonsils, and adenoids) to aggressive lymphomas. It is a complication of immunosuppression and is usually caused by Epstein-Barr virus (EBV) infection leading to B-cell (more common) or T-cell proliferation. Presentation is highly variable, including lymphadenopathy, fever, weight loss, tonsillar enlargement, gastrointestinal symptoms (diarrhea, vomiting, anorexia, abdominal pain), and rarely central nervous system symptoms. Fulminant disease can present as a mononucleosis-like illness followed by sepsis, disseminated intravascular coagulation, and multisystem organ failure. Excisional biopsy, CT scans, and bone marrow aspiration are done for staging. Treatment modalities include reduction of immunosuppression, local control with surgery and/or radiotherapy, rituximab (a monoclonal antibody that inhibits B-cell proliferation), chemotherapy, and antiviral agents.

Preoperative assessment should focus on the transplanted organ function, signs of rejection, current and recent infections, and evaluation for the following chemotherapy and immunosuppressant side effects:

- Cyclosporine: nephrotoxicity, hepatotoxicity, neurotoxicity, hypertension, hirsutism, gum hyperplasia
- Tacrolimus: nephrotoxicity, pancreatitis/diabetes, hypertension, hypertrophic cardiomyopathy

- Azathioprine: myelosuppression, hepatotoxicity
- Steroids: hypertension, diabetes, neurotoxicity

ANESTHETIC MANAGEMENT

- Continue all preoperative immunosuppressant agents.
- Use antibiotic prophylaxis and aseptic technique to prevent infection.
- Make a careful assessment of the airway and preparation for upper airway obstruction, including oral airways, laryngeal mask airway, and possibly preinduction IV placement.
- If stridor is present, involvement of the epiglottis and trachea may be present. Spontaneous ventilation should be maintained, and advanced airway equipment such as rigid bronchoscopy should be available.
- If vomiting and diarrhea are present, ensure adequate hydration and consider a rapid-sequence induction.
- Cyclosporine can potentiate the effect of succinylcholine. Azathioprine can antagonize the effect of nondepolarizing muscle relaxants; however, the level of antagonism is probably clinically insignificant. As these drug interactions can be variable, twitch monitoring should be used.
- Post-heart transplant patients have denervated hearts, causing a lack of a heart rate (HR) response to hypotension/hypertension, hypovolemia, light anesthesia, opioids, and atropine, as these are all mediated by the autonomic nervous system. Direct-acting medications such as epinephrine, norepinephrine, dopamine, and isoproterenol will cause an increase in HR, cardiac output, and blood pressure.
- A five-lead electrocardiogram should be continuously monitored for heart transplant patients, as they are at risk for post transplant coronary artery disease, leading to perioperative myocardial infarction and arrhythmias. A double P wave may be noted, one from the remnant sinoatrial node that is not conducted.

POSTOPERATIVE CONSIDERATIONS

If severe airway obstruction or sleep apnea was present, the patient should be recovered in the intensive care unit setting and observed overnight. Mild to moderate sleep apnea patients can be monitored in the postanesthesia care unit.

DOs and DON'Ts

✓ Do minimize the number of lines placed and attempt to take out unnecessary lines postoperatively to avoid infection.

⊗ Do not perform a nasal intubation unless absolutely necessary, given that nasal flora may be a potential source of infection.

(continued)

✓   Do ensure adequate IV access and adequate volume replacement, as the transplanted heart is preload dependent.
✓   Do carefully assess renal function before considering nonsteroidal anti-inflammatory drugs for postoperative pain. They may act synergistically with immunosuppressive agents to impair renal function.
⊗   Do not administer rectal acetaminophen, as this may lead to infection or visceral perforation. Hepatic function should be assessed before oral acetaminophen is used.

FACTOID

In children, PTLD is the most common posttransplant malignancy. Risk factors include younger age, primary EBV infection, EBV seropositive donor to an EBV seronegative recipient, and higher cumulative dose of immunosuppression. Incidence of PTLD varies by the type of solid organ transplanted: kidney 1%-10%, liver 4%-15%, heart and lung 6%-20%.

49 SICKLE CELL DISEASE

Caleb Ing, MD, MS

YOUR PATIENT

A 13-year-old girl in her usual state of health presents from home with a history of hemoglobin SS (HbSS) for laparoscopic cholecystectomy. The patient has had a history of multiple sickle cell crises, with her most recent episode of acute chest syndrome occurring 6 months ago.

Laboratory: Hematocrit is 26.

PREOPERATIVE CONSIDERATIONS

Sickle cell disease results from an inherited structural disorder of the hemoglobin β-globin chain. There is a wide range of severity and speed of progression, with clinical consequences ranging from benign sickle trait to severe symptomatology in homozygous HbSS patients. Patients with severe disease may have a history of chronic hemolytic anemia, frequent vaso-occlusive crises, and chronic organ damage, including cardiomegaly, pulmonary hypertension, and ischemic strokes. These patients are at higher risk for perioperative complications.

HbSS patients are at risk of having their red blood cells form distorted sickle cells when the patient is exposed to hypoxia; this is exacerbated by acidosis, dehydration, or hypothermia with vasoconstriction. Hypoxia with a PaO_2 below 40-50 mm Hg typically results in the formation of sickle cells, but sickling can be seen even in well-oxygenated SS cells. Increased age or the presence of infection can also increase the risk of sickling.

Preoperative transfusion regimens range from aggressive (lowering the HbS to less than 30%), to conservative (correcting only the anemia), to not transfusing at all. Some studies have shown that for low- to moderate-risk procedures, maintaining a Hb of 10 g/dL results in no outcome differences from a more aggressive technique and has the added benefit of reducing transfusion-related complications. As a result, the trend in perioperative transfusions has been moving toward a more conservative approach. The decision to transfuse, however, needs to be made based on the risk factors of each individual patient, and consultation with a hematologist is recommended for complicated patients. The crossmatching of blood for patients who have had multiple transfusions may be a problem, and blood availability should be addressed prior to the start of surgery. An additional consideration is that preoperative medications that can depress spontaneous ventilation should be used with caution and supplemental oxygen should be considered.

In the case of this child, a blood transfusion would be recommended as well as a consultation with the patient's hematologist to determine her baseline hematocrit and transfusion goals.

ANESTHETIC MANAGEMENT

- Anesthetic goals include maintaining oxygenation and normothermia while avoiding hypovolemia, acidosis, infection, and stasis.
- The use of tourniquets for orthopedic surgery is controversial, and the risk of precipitating an acute event must be weighed against the benefit of decreased bleeding.
- Controversy exists over the use of general versus regional anesthesia, with some studies showing worsened outcomes with regional anesthesia, while others show no difference.
- In cases requiring contrast dye, the use of hypertonic dye has been thought to induce sickling, so isotonic contrast is a safer alternative. Induced hypothermia for cardiopulmonary bypass can potentially precipitate vaso-occlusive crisis, but it has been performed safely.

POSTOPERATIVE CONSIDERATIONS

Patients should be observed for postoperative pain, pulmonary compromise, and hypovolemia. Early mobilization with aggressive chest physiotherapy is recommended. Supplemental oxygen should be weaned slowly, as abrupt withdrawal has been anecdotally associated with vaso-occlusive crises.

DOs and DON'Ts

✓ Do get a detailed history focusing on the history of crises and chronic end-organ damage.

✓ Do maintain oxygenation and normothermia and avoid hypovolemia, acidosis, infection, and stasis.

✓ Do consult with a hematologist to make decisions concerning transfusions for complicated patients.

⊗ Do not adopt an aggressive transfusion protocol by lowering the HbS <30% for every patient.

CONTROVERSIES

- Perioperative blood transfusion
- Regional versus general anesthesia

SURGICAL CONCERNS

A discussion with the surgical team regarding the potential for blood loss and the need for blood products for this case is needed.

FACTOID

Patients who develop acute chest syndrome (ACS) present with fever, cough, tachypnea, pleuritic chest pain, hypoxemia, pulmonary hypertension, and radiological evidence of lung infiltrates. ACS is responsible for up to 25% of sickle cell–related deaths. It has a postoperative incidence as high as 10% and on average develops 3 days after surgery.

50 MASSIVE TRANSFUSION

Manon Haché, MD

YOUR PATIENT

An 11-year-old, 30-kg patient presents to the operating room emergently after being hit by a car. He was unconscious at the scene and intubated. He was volume resuscitated and so far has received 40 mL/kg of lactated Ringer's and 2 units of blood. He remains hemodynamically unstable (heart rate 130, blood pressure 80/35) and has a positive focused assessment with sonography for trauma exam. His head CT scan reveals diffuse edema with no focal bleeding. His cervical spine CT is unremarkable, and he remains in a cervical collar. The plan is to do an exploratory laparotomy for control of bleeding.

PREOPERATIVE CONSIDERATIONS

Trauma is the leading cause of death in children between 1 and 18 years old. We consider adult patients to have received a massive transfusion when they have received 10 units of blood; in children, several definitions have been used, including >40 or >70 mL/kg.

Recently, adult trauma literature has shown that using a fixed ratio of blood products (1:1:1 PRBC:FFP:plt [packed red blood cells:fresh frozen plasma:platelets) may improve outcomes. This is starting to be applied to pediatric patients, although the mechanism responsible for massive blood loss can be different (ie, more blunt trauma in pediatric patients).

This patient also has a significant head trauma, and his blood pressure should be kept at a level that will ensure adequate cerebral perfusion. An intracranial pressure monitor would be helpful to guide ideal cerebral perfusion pressure.

ANESTHETIC MANAGEMENT

- Warm the room.
- Be ready for transfusion with fluid warmer and blood infusion set; get two large-bore peripheral IVs. Arterial access is desirable but secondary.
- Ensure that the blood bank is sending adequate amounts of blood products.

- Consider activating the massive transfusion protocol if present when >40 mL/kg blood loss is anticipated.
- Give fresh frozen plasma (FFP) and platelets early (ratio close to 1:1:1).
- Cryoprecipitate (4 mL/kg) should be given to maintain fibrinogen above 1 g/L or for ongoing bleeding after giving one round of PRBC/FFP/plt.
- Be ready for significant hemodynamic compromise with the laparotomy.
- Calcium levels should be followed and repleted with transfusion.

POSTOPERATIVE CONSIDERATIONS

Occasionally, the source of bleeding will not be able to be determined, and damage control resuscitation is necessary. This involves packing the abdomen and correcting coagulopathy, acidosis, and hypothermia before going back for a second look.

DOs and DON'Ts

✓ Do warm the operating room and all blood products, as hypothermia is common and will contribute to coagulopathy.
✓ Do use a rapid infusion device.
⊗ Do not wait to activate the massive transfusion protocol if significant bleeding is anticipated.
✓ Do use FFP and platelets early.
✓ Do not forget to replete calcium, 10 mg/kg to maintain ionized calcium above 1 mmol/L.

CONTROVERSIES

- The "perfect" ratio of blood products to be transfused is not yet known, but there is evidence that giving FFP early can be beneficial, given that a lot of trauma victims present to the emergency room with a coagulopathy related to trauma, even before receiving multiple transfusions of crystalloids and blood products.
- Tranexamic acid (1 g over 10 minutes, then 1 g over 8 hours) has been shown to decrease bleeding in adult trauma when given early (within 3 hours).
- Factor VII has also been advocated for uncontrolled bleeding; standard dosing is 90 µg/kg.

FACTOID

Historically, "bloodletting" was thought to be effective for treating a multitude of diseases, to rid patients of "bad humors." Syncope was often considered beneficial, and many phlebotomies would not end until the patient started to feel faint.

51 METHEMOGLOBINEMIA

Teeda Pinyavat, MD

YOUR PATIENT

A 4-year-old undergoes an uneventful esophagogastroduodenoscopy (EGD) but is noted to be cyanotic in the postanesthesia care unit 1 hour later. He appears agitated and tachypneic, and has perioral cyanosis. Despite being placed on 100% oxygen by face mask, his SaO$_2$ is 86%. His lungs are clear, and his stat chest x-ray is normal. An arterial blood sample is chocolate-colored. PaO$_2$ and calculated oxygen saturation are normal. Cetacaine spray (14% benzocaine, 2% butamben, 2% tetracaine) was used for topicalization.

PREOPERATIVE CONSIDERATIONS

Patients at higher risk of symptomatic methemoglobinemia include children less than 4 months of age; patients with methemoglobin reductase deficiency (more likely in Native Americans of Alaska or Inuit descent), G6PD deficiency, or cardiopulmonary disease; and elderly and anemic patients.

There should be high suspicion for methemoglobinemia in a cyanotic patient who has been exposed to any of the following: nitrates (nitroglycerin, nitric oxide, nitroprusside, silver nitrate, metoclopramide), local anesthetics (benzocaine, prilocaine, lidocaine, EMLA cream), sulfonamides (antimalarials, primaquine, chloroquine), dapsone, and acetaminophen.

Manifestations vary by level of methemoglobin (metHb): cyanosis at 10%; headache, shortness of breath, weakness, fatigue, confusion, tachypnea, and tachycardia at 30%-50%; coma, seizures, arrhythmia, and acidosis at >50%; and fatality at >70%.

ANESTHETIC MANAGEMENT

- Rule out other causes of cyanosis, including airway, pulmonary, and cardiac.
- The pulse oximeter reading plateaus at around 85% when metHb levels are 30% or greater. MetHb absorbs the two wavelengths 660 nm (red) and 940 nm (infrared) in equal amounts, and this results in the

calculated saturation of 85%, although this number does not reflect the true oxygen saturation.

- Check arterial blood gases. The PaO_2 should be high or normal because metHb does not affect the amount of oxygen dissolved in the blood. For the same reason, calculated oxygen saturation is reported as normal because this is calculated from the PaO_2.
- Check a true oxygen saturation using co-oximetry. Co-oximetry uses four wavelengths and is able to differentiate metHb, carboxyHb, oxyHb, and deoxyHb.
- MetHb levels >20% should prompt treatment including elimination of the causative agent, maximizing oxygen delivery, and giving methylene blue 1-2 mg/kg IV over 5 minutes (can repeat in 1 hour if the patient is still symptomatic; maximum dose 7 mg/kg).
- Methylene blue also leads to artifacts in the pulse oximetry reading (as low as 65%) due to its absorbance of light in the red range.
- Resolution of methemoglobinemia usually occurs within 20-60 minutes after administration of methylene blue.

POSTOPERATIVE CONSIDERATIONS

Rebound methemoglobinemia can occur up to 20 hours after treatment. Therefore, close observation is warranted and overnight admission should be considered.

DOs and DON'Ts

✓ Do consider metHb early when a high PaO_2 is combined with a low SaO_2.

✓ Do quickly send off a sample for co-oximetry, on ice, before initiating treatment, as methylene blue alters the results of co-oximetry.

⊗ Do not delay treatment for co-oximetry results.

⊗ Do not treat with methylene blue if the patient has G6PD deficiency. In these patients, methylene blue will be ineffective, will paradoxically increase metHb levels, and can lead to red blood cell hemolysis. For these patients, exchange transfusion, vitamin C, or hyperbaric oxygen should be considered.

⊗ Do not give methylene blue if metHb levels are <20% or give more than 7 mg/kg, as it can paradoxically increase metHb levels as much as 10%.

✓ Do know that the average dose delivered in a benzocaine spray is 56 mg, although it is very difficult to predict benzocaine delivery and absorption. Doses as low as 3-5 mg/kg have been associated with methemoglobinemia.

CONTROVERSIES

The routine use of benzocaine sprays for EGD, transesophageal echocardiography, and bronchoscopy has come into question. In 2006, the Veterans Administration system announced that it would stop using benzocaine for mouth and throat procedures.

FACTOIDS

- The Food and Drug Administration also warns against benzocaine usage in children under age 2, after reports of methemoglobinemia from the use of benzocaine gel in teething children.
- In a retrospective review of 138 cases of acquired methemoglobinemia, the most common causes were dapsone (42%), benzocaine (4%), and primaquine (4%). The most severe cases were caused by HurriCaine spray (20% benzocaine).
- The incidence of methemoglobinemia after benzocaine is reportedly 1 in 7000 exposures.

52 HEPARIN-INDUCED THROMBOCYTOPENIA

Caleb Ing, MD, MS

YOUR PATIENT

A 12-year-old boy with a history of double-outlet right ventricle who has had an initial surgery for a Blalock-Taussig shunt and then a repair with placement of a right ventricle–to–pulmonary artery (RV-to-PA) conduit now presents with increasing shortness of breath for replacement of his RV-to-PA conduit. Of note, during his prior procedure, he developed severe thrombocytopenia and was found to have heparin-induced thrombocytopenia (HIT) antibodies.

PREOPERATIVE CONSIDERATIONS

Heparin-induced thrombocytopenia occurs in two forms. Type I thrombocytopenia results in a mild, transient reduction of platelets, acts by a nonimmunologic mechanism, and occurs 24-72 hours after heparin therapy. The more serious Type II thrombocytopenia, which is also known as heparin-associated thrombocytopenia and thrombosis (HITT), is immunologically mediated, occurs 5-10 days after heparin exposure, and results in marked thrombocytopenia with the potential for severe thromboembolic complications. The more serious thrombocytopenia and thrombosis reactions can be life-threatening. This case refers only to Type II HIT.

A complex of heparin and platelet factor 4 (PF4) activates this immunologic response. When this heparin-PF4 complex binds to an activated platelet surface, it results in further platelet activation and release of PF4, resulting in a vicious cycle of platelet activation and aggregation leading to thrombocytopenia and thrombosis.

Diagnosis for HIT is typically made on clinical grounds (platelet drop of 50% or new thrombosis 5-10 days after initiating heparin therapy), since testing typically has a slow turnaround time. The gold standard for confirmation of HIT is the 14C-serotonin release assay; however, because of the expense and difficulty in obtaining the test, an ELISA immunoassay is the more common test that is performed. The ELISA test is very sensitive to heparin-PF4 antibodies, so a negative test strongly suggests the absence of HIT, but a positive test has unclear clinical implications. Decisions on the likelihood of HIT must be made based on a pretest clinical score (the 4 Ts: thrombocytopenia, timing of platelet fall, thrombosis, and other causes for thrombocytopenia).

The decision to use heparin for anticoagulation during cardiopulmonary bypass (CPB) is dependent on whether circulating heparin-PF4 antibodies are still detectable. HIT antibodies typically disappear after a period of 50-90 days. If HIT antibodies are no longer present, unfractionated heparin (UFH) can be used for CPB. In cases where IgG antibodies to heparin-PF4 remain, a more specific functional assay such as the serotonin release assay or a platelet aggregation assay can be used. If these assays are either positive for HIT or unavailable, an alternative anticoagulant can be used, or heparin can be attempted after intraoperative plasma exchange to reduce the antibody titer.

In the case of this child, an immunoassay for HIT antibodies could be undertaken to determine the correct course of action.

ANESTHETIC MANAGEMENT

- All forms of heparin should be avoided to prevent the development of thrombosis.
- If intraoperative anticoagulation is necessary, potential nonheparin anticoagulants include bivalirudin, argatroban, and lepirudin. Although all three of these agents have been safely used in children, no formal pediatric pharmacokinetic or efficacy studies have been performed with lepirudin.

POSTOPERATIVE CONSIDERATIONS

Heparin should be avoided in patients with a history of HIT requiring postoperative anticoagulation.

DOs and DON'Ts

✓   Do get a detailed history focusing on prior thrombocytopenia episodes and resulting laboratory studies.
✓   Do repeat a HIT immunoassay to aid in decision making.

CONTROVERSIES

Nonheparin anticoagulant vs heparin with plasma exchange in patients with unclear risk for HIT.

SURGICAL CONCERNS

A discussion should occur with the surgical team about the potential for additional blood loss when using a nonheparin anticoagulant that cannot be easily reversed, as well as parameters for monitoring anticoagulation.

FACTOID

The incidence of HIT antibody after UFH use during cardiac surgery ranges from 1.7%-6%, with 50% of children testing positive for the antibody after reoperations. Only 1.3%, however, develop clinical symptoms.

PART 7

GASTROINTESTINAL DISEASES

53 ESOPHAGOGASTRO-DUODENOSCOPY

Philipp J. Houck, MD

YOUR PATIENT

An 8-year-old presents for esophagogastroduodenoscopy (EGD) for gastroesophageal reflux disease (GERD).

PREOPERATIVE CONSIDERATIONS

Gastroesophageal reflux disease is one of the most common comorbidities in our field. It is more prevalent in patients with neurologic impairment, obesity, repaired esophageal atresia or other congenital esophageal diseases, and cystic fibrosis. GER is a normal physiologic process that occurs several times per day in healthy infants, children, and adults. GERD is present when the reflux of gastric contents causes troublesome symptoms and/or complications. Patients may present with asthma, bronchopulmonary dysplasia, or apparent life-threatening events that may be related to pulmonary aspiration.

ANESTHETIC MANAGEMENT

- Rapid-sequence induction, which has its own risks in pediatric anesthesia, may be necessary.
- If pulmonary aspiration is not a leading concern (ie, symptoms are not severe and are mostly postprandial) and the patient is school-aged, tracheal intubation can be avoided and a total intravenous anesthesia technique can be used, with supplemental oxygen being supplied through a nasal cannula.
- In smaller children, a mask induction and endotracheal intubation is the most practical choice. This allows insertion and manipulation of the endoscope without impeding the patency of the airway.
- The most stimulating part of this procedure is the insertion of the endoscope. To facilitate the insertion of the endoscope in the esophagus, the head can be flexed while the patient is in left lateral position.

POSTOPERATIVE CONSIDERATIONS

In infants, prolonged insufflation and the use of high insufflation pressures can lead to a distended abdomen that may impede ventilation. Intestinal perforation can present with a similar picture.

DOs and DON'Ts

- ✓ Do flex the head during the insertion of the scope.
- ✓ Do choose a rapid-sequence induction in patients with severe GERD, particularly when the patient regurgitates food even after adequate fasting.
- ⊗ Do not use high insufflation pressures in infants.
- ✓ Do intubate young children.

CONTROVERSIES

Topicalization of the larynx may decrease the incidence of laryngospasm during insertion of the endoscope, but it results in an unprotected airway during and after emergence from anesthesia.

SURGICAL CONCERNS

The incidence of intestinal perforation is low (0.1%). Signs of a perforation are an unusually distended abdomen, abdominal pain, fever, and subcutaneous or mediastinal air. Injuries during an EGD in a stable patient without peritonitis can be managed conservatively; colonic perforation during a sigmoidoscopy requires immediate surgical repair.

FACTOID

More than 25% of adults in the United States use antisecretory medications at least 3 times per month.

54 CONTROL OF UPPER GASTROINTESTINAL BLEEDING

Manon Haché, MD

YOUR PATIENT

A 10-year-old presented to the emergency room after having emesis of bright red blood 3 times. Hematocrit on admission was 15. The patient received 20 mL/kg of packed red blood cells and was booked for an emergency diagnostic esophagogastroduodenoscopy with banding of varices. Pertinent past medical history reveals that he was diagnosed at age 6 months with cystic fibrosis (CF). He has had banding of esophageal varices 3 times in the past. He also has chronic lung disease requiring chest physical therapy (PT), a cough assist vest, inhaled tobramycin, and DNase, fluticasone, and albuterol inhalers. He just finished a course of IV antibiotics last week for increased pulmonary secretions and presumed pneumonia.

PREOPERATIVE CONSIDERATIONS

Upper gastrointestinal bleeding can originate from any area proximal to the ligament of Treitz. Most commonly, any bleeding that occurs distally will present as melena. The most common differential diagnosis of upper gastrointestinal bleeding in children includes gastritis, peptic ulcer disease, Mallory-Weiss syndrome, and esophageal varices. Given this patient's history, the most likely cause is variceal bleeding.

Cystic fibrosis is a genetic disorder associated with chronic lung disease and pancreatic insufficiency. Pulmonary disease is responsible for more than 90% of the morbidity in these patients. Classically, patients are diagnosed by performing a sweat test. Chloride in sweat will be markedly increased. These patients can present at birth with meconium ileus with rare perforation. They may also present with severe pulmonary manifestations; thick secretions or mucus plugs, leading to multiple infections; or severe persistent episodes of obstructive airway disease. This may eventually lead to pulmonary hypertension and cor pulmonale. They may also present with malnutrition or diabetes resulting from exocrine or endocrine pancreatic dysfunction. They may also present with liver cirrhosis. They can develop upper gastrointestinal bleeding from esophageal varices secondary to portal hypertension and also have coagulopathy from liver failure or cirrhosis and malnutrition.

ANESTHETIC MANAGEMENT

- Thoroughly assess the severity of pulmonary disease in order to better plan intraoperative and postoperative management; oxygen should be available as well as biphasic positive airway pressure if it is used preoperatively
- Humidify gases. Frequent suctioning or lavage of secretions may be necessary.
- Assess the degree of pancreatic involvement and manage diabetes if present; frequent blood glucose monitoring is indicated.
- Sinus involvement may act as a bacterial reservoir and also trigger bronchospasm.
- Upper gastrointestinal bleeding may be severe, and adequate volume resuscitation as well as preparation for possible blood transfusion should be made.
- Manage coagulopathy, if present.
- Have blood products available.

POSTOPERATIVE CONSIDERATIONS

Early extubation should be the goal with all CF patients, as prolonged intubation may increase morbidity and mortality. Early chest PT and mobilization should be encouraged.

DOs and DON'Ts

- ✓ Do get a good sense of baseline pulmonary function in CF patients.
- ✓ Do make sure that the patient has been adequately volume resuscitated.
- ⊗ Do not forget about pancreatic involvement.
- ✓ Do a rapid-sequence induction and have two suctions available in case one clots.
- ✓ Do plan for early extubation and chest PT if possible.

CONTROVERSIES

The risk of bleeding when banding esophageal varices electively (without recent bleeding) is very low. These patients may be managed without endotracheal intubation.

SURGICAL CONCERNS

In CF patients, it may be hard to distinguish massive upper gastrointestinal bleeding from hemoptysis. These patients may have a bronchiectasis that causes massive hemoptysis and requires bronchial artery embolization.

FACTOID

The gene causing CF was identified in 1989, but so far gene therapy has not proven successful. There are more than 1000 genetic mutations that have been identified.

55 LIVER BIOPSY

Manon Haché, MD

YOUR PATIENT

A 2-month-old female infant with persistent jaundice is scheduled for a liver biopsy. She was born at 35 weeks' gestation.

Laboratory findings: Total bilirubin 10.3; conjugated 6.0; international normalized ratio 1.25; partial thromboplastin time 32; albumin 20.

PREOPERATIVE CONSIDERATIONS

Physiologic unconjugated hyperbilirubinemia is very common and occurs in about two-thirds of newborns. It usually becomes apparent on day 2 or 3 of life and lasts around 10 days. Persistent or severe hyperbilirubinemia warrants further evaluation. It can result from increased bilirubin production, deficiency of hepatic uptake, defects of conjugation, and increased enterohepatic circulation. Increased values of conjugated bilirubin warrant a cholestasis workup to evaluate for biliary atresia. Time is of the essence because the success of the Kasai procedure is thought to be better when it is performed early, preferably before 3 months of age.

ANESTHETIC MANAGEMENT

- Use general anesthesia without an endotracheal tube.
- Sevoflurane mask induction and maintenance or propofol can be used.
- Use opioids judiciously; the surgery is not very painful, but patients are expected to remain flat for a prolonged period postoperatively. Fentanyl 1-2 µg/kg is a good choice.

POSTOPERATIVE CONSIDERATIONS

Patients must remain in the postanesthesia care unit for 4 hours for monitoring of possible hemodynamic consequences of bleeding at the site of the liver biopsy; they must take nothing by mouth for the first 2 hours.

DOs and DON'Ts

✓ Do perform brief general anesthesia. Patients must remain absolutely still.

✓ Do be prepared for significant bleeding. Have an active type and cross.

⊗ If possible, do not delay surgery.

✓ Do keep an IV in place in case bleeding develops later.

CONTROVERSIES

Tylenol administration (10 mg/kg) is most likely fine for patients with hyperbilirubinemia without liver failure.

SURGICAL CONCERNS

Guidance of the needle biopsy is by percussion or ultrasound, especially for patients with transplanted livers. There is a small risk of significant bleeding, less so with transplanted livers, because of adhesions to surrounding structures.

FACTOID

The implementation of stool color cards in Taiwan in 2004 helped increase the number of patients diagnosed and treated with the Kasai operation before age 3 months.

56 LIVER TRANSPLANTATION

Philipp J. Houck, MD

YOUR PATIENT

A 2-year-old patient with biliary atresia presents with portal hypertension, esophageal varices, and massive ascites for liver transplantation after a failed Kasai procedure.

Laboratory findings: International normalized ratio 4.2; total bilirubin 16.

PREOPERATIVE CONSIDERATIONS

Biliary atresia is the most common indication for pediatric liver transplantation. Up to 20% of patients have other congenital malformations, including splenic malformations, situs inversus, or absence of the inferior vena cava. After diagnosis in infancy, a Kasai portoenterostomy (a Roux-en-Y loop is anastomosed to exposed ductules at the surface of the porta hepatis), which corrects hyperbilirubinemia within 6 months if successful, is the standard of care. This has to be performed before 3 months of age, and the failure rate is high. Those patients develop portal fibrosis, cirrhosis, and portal hypertension. Patients may have the usual stigmata of liver failure and can be hypervolemic, hyperdynamic, and coagulopathic.

ANESTHETIC MANAGEMENT

- Use rapid-sequence induction for patients with a full stomach or massive ascites; use a cuffed endotracheal tube.
- Arterial line and central venous access must be obtained above the diaphragm because of interruption of blood flow from the aorta and the inferior vena cava during cross-clamping.
- Assess arterial blood gases, hemoglobin, and urine output hourly. Every 2 hours determine complete blood cell count, coagulation factors, and fibrinogen.
- Avoid hypothermia.
- Preanhepatic phase: Prepare patient for caval cross-clamp, including optimizing hemodynamics with volume (central venous pressure

should be >10) and inotropic and or vasopressor infusions, making sure patient is not acidotic or hyperkalemic (bicarbonate, furosemide, hyperventilation as needed).

- Anhepatic phase: There is little caval blood flow with caval cross-clamping in patients without collaterals; therefore, it is better tolerated in patients with chronic portal hypertension. Piggyback technique preserves caval blood flow but may require a caval cross-clamp on short notice.
- Postanhepatic phase: Reperfusion of the graft will lead to acidemia, hyperkalemia, and hypothermia. Prepare for unclamping with hyperventilation, give calcium and $NaHCO_3$, and have insulin, glucose, and epinephrine available. To maintain patency of the hepatic artery, it may be necessary to start a heparin infusion. After anastomosis of the hepatic artery and portal vein, the bile duct will be anastomosed, or in patients with a prior Kasai procedure, the Roux-en-Y limb can be used for bile drainage.

POSTOPERATIVE CONSIDERATIONS

Defer extubation in most patients, particularly when the abdominal wall was not closed or reexploration is planned. In patients with large grafts, abdominal compartment syndrome must be treated promptly to avoid abdominal ischemia and high airway pressures, which may lead to hemodynamic compromise. Graft-related problem in the early postoperative phase are vascular complications, biliary complications, or allograft rejection.

DOs and DON'Ts

✓ Do have sufficient amounts of blood products available at all times.
⊗ Do not use lactated Ringer's solution because patients cannot metabolize lactate.
✓ Do have a large central venous line in the internal jugular or subclavian vein.
⊗ Do not overcorrect the coagulopathy.
✓ Do be restrictive with platelet transfusions.
✓ Do communicate clearly with the surgeon regarding cross-clamping.

CONTROVERSIES

In some centers, thromboelastography is used to help guide management of coagulopathy.

SURGICAL CONCERNS

Hepatic artery thrombosis is a constant threat. Usually no platelets are given until the platelet count is very low; avoid overcorrection of coagulopathy for the same reason.

Avoid high central venous pressure after the reperfusion, since this may lead to swelling of the liver.

FACTOID

In 1955, Kasai did not find a bile duct in a 3-month-old girl, which made her condition biliary atresia of a type that was not correctable at the time. In desperation, he made an incision at the porta hepatis and placed the duodenum over the region. She drained bile in her stool, and the Kasai procedure was born.

57 CROHN'S DISEASE

Philipp J. Houck, MD

YOUR PATIENT

A 16-year-old patient with a known history of Crohn's disease presents with an anal fistula. He has had two prior bowel resections.

PREOPERATIVE CONSIDERATIONS

Crohn's disease is a chronic inflammation of the gastrointestinal tract with an incidence of 7 in 100,000. The disease can occur anywhere from the mouth to the anus, but it usually involves the ileum and colon. Patients present with abdominal pain, vomiting (which can be constant), diarrhea, and weight loss. Rectal fistulas are common. A combination of antibiotics, immunomodulators, and biologic agents as well as conservative operative procedures are used to treat the fistulas.

The chronic inflammation and hemorrhage may lead to anemia. Albumin loss through diseased mucosa can lead to hypoalbuminemia. Malnutrition can be severe enough to require total parental nutrition. Evaluate the intravascular fluid and electrolyte status, particularly after the patient receives a bowel preparation. Ankylosing spondylitis and Crohn's disease are both caused by the HLA-B27 genotype, and some patients have both diseases. In patients with ankylosing spondylitis, a direct laryngoscopy can be difficult.

Patients can be very apprehensive about the prospect of multiple bowel resections.

Children on azathioprine or 6-mercaptopurine can have leukopenia and drug-induced hepatitis.

ANESTHETIC MANAGEMENT

- Neuroaxial anesthesia is theoretically a good choice. Most 16-year-old patients prefer to be unconscious during a perianal procedure. The incidence of postdural puncture headache decreases with age, which changes the risk-benefit ratio in young patients with a low risk for cardiac or cerebral complications to favor general anesthesia.
- General anesthesia with either total intravenous anesthesia with a nasal canula or laryngeal mask airway may be considered, but positioning of

the patient in a lithotomy and steep Trendelenburg position may require endotracheal intubation.

- Avoid acetaminophen in patients with concomitant liver disease.
- Give a stress dose if the patient is taking steroids or has taken them in the past 6 months.
- Patients who take infliximab (a monoclonal antibody used for fistula closure or maintenance therapy) are at risk of an acute coronary syndrome; postoperative muscle weakness has been reported.

POSTOPERATIVE CONSIDERATIONS

Patients with Crohn's disease usually have chronic abdominal pain, and their postoperative pain may be difficult to control. Consider using a multimodal approach and utilize complementary methods.

DOs and DON'Ts

✓   Do use the patient's indwelling permanent access, if present.
⊗   Do not give nitrous oxide.
⊗   Do not give paralytics if stimulation of the sphincter muscle is planned.

CONTROVERSIES

Surgical site infections in colorectal surgery may be decreased by hyperoxia. Classically, papers quote using a fraction of inspired oxygen of 80%.

SURGICAL CONCERNS

Surgical treatment of skin tags in this population, whether conservative or aggressive, is associated with prohibitive morbidity.

FACTOID

Smoking may increase the risk of Crohn's disease.

PART 8

METABOLIC DISEASES

58 EGG AND SOY ALLERGY

Manon Haché, MD

YOUR PATIENT

A 10-year-old girl with chronic abdominal pain is presenting for an upper endoscopy and biopsies because of abdominal pain. She has multiple allergies, including penicillin, soy, eggs, and nuts, all causing anaphylaxis. She has never required general anesthesia before.

PREOPERATIVE CONSIDERATIONS

Patients with multiple allergies may be at risk for allergies to any product they come in contact with. In particular, propofol is manufactured with soy oil and egg lecithin/phosphatide, and there are concerns regarding its use in children with egg and soy allergies. It is unlikely that patients who are able to tolerate cooked eggs will react to propofol, as the heating process may denature some of the allergenic proteins, and this may also be the case during propofol manufacturing. There are only two published cases of patients with egg allergy who have suffered an allergic reaction to propofol, and most documented cases of propofol allergy were to the isopropyl or phenol group rather than the lipid vehicle. That being said, the package inserts in Australia and the United Kingdom list allergies as relative contraindication to the use of propofol (egg/soy in Australia, soy/peanut in the United Kingdom).

ANESTHETIC MANAGEMENT

- Propofol may be used.
- If you choose to avoid propofol, you have multiple options: Sevoflurane induction and maintenance after endotracheal intubation, midazolam/ketamine/dexmedetomidine combinations (midazolam 0.1 mg/kg; ketamine 1 mg/kg/dose, titrate to effect; dexmedetomidine 0.2-0.5 mcg/kg/h).
- There is no evidence that pretreatment with antihistamines or corticosteroids will prevent allergic reactions in patients with severe allergies.

POSTOPERATIVE CONSIDERATIONS

Be aware of your patient's risk for allergic reactions and ensure her return to baseline before discharging her home.

DOs and DON'Ts

- ✓ Do be aware that egg allergy is not a contraindication to the use of propofol.
- ✓ Do know that there are plenty of suitable alternatives should you choose to avoid propofol.
- ⊗ Do not premedicate patients with allergies to avoid allergic reactions.
- ✓ Do keep anaphylaxis in mind in any patient presenting with bronchospasm and hypotension.

CONTROVERSIES

Despite the product being the same, manufactured by the same company, package inserts for Diprivan 10% in Australia and the United Kingdom list food allergies as a relative contraindication to the use of propofol (egg/soy in Australia, soy/peanut in the United Kingdom), while there are no such warnings in the United States.

FACTOID

The first documented anaphylactic death occurred in 2641 BC when Menes, an Egyptian pharaoh, died after a wasp or bee sting.

59 HYPERKALEMIA

Radhika Dinavahi

YOUR PATIENT

An 8-year-old child presents with a history of end-stage renal disease (ESRD) from glomerulonephritis. He is not dialysis dependent, and he comes to the operating room for a nonscheduled renal transplant.

Laboratory findings: K 7.5; HCO_3 14
Electrocardiogram (ECG): Peaked T waves in all leads

PREOPERATIVE CONSIDERATIONS

Chronic renal failure in children has a prevalence of about 18-58 cases per million children. The incidence is equal in both sexes, although obstructive uropathies are more common in males.

- Although the potassium may be chronically elevated in chronic kidney disease, this presentation is notable for the cardiac abnormality noted on ECG. Because of this finding, one should be concerned and make an effort to decrease the potassium prior to induction of anesthesia.
- The bicarbonate level is also chronically low in kidney disease due to metabolic acidosis. The patient is probably taking supplemental bicarbonate at home, and this should be given not only to treat the acidosis, but also to help promote intracellular movement of potassium and treat the hyperkalemia.

ANESTHETIC MANAGEMENT

- Hyperkalemia is treated with insulin, dextrose, and sodium bicarbonate prior to arrival at the operating room.
- Administer dextrose 1 g/kg IV over 15 minutes with 0.2 unit insulin/kg.
- Administer calcium chloride 4-5 mg/kg IV over 5-10 minutes to stabilize cardiac membrane.
- Administer 1 mEq/kg of sodium bicarbonate over 10 minutes.
- Kayexalate administered rectally has faster activity than oral. Administer Kayexalate 1 g/kg rectally every 2 hours as needed.
- Consider furosemide administration and/or albuterol treatment.
- Repeat potassium and ECG after therapy to monitor for resolution.

- General anesthesia may reduce renal blood flow in up to 50% of patients, so remain cautious in patients with renal insufficiency.
- The function of cholinesterase may be impaired, resulting in a prolonged effect of succinylcholine if it is used in patients with ESRD. Caution with succinylcholine use is particularly indicated where potassium is elevated, as succinylcholine transiently exacerbates hyperkalemia.
- Consider normal saline usage for IV hydration given decreased potassium content.
- Use fentanyl and hydromorphone for opioids. Avoid morphine, as its metabolites remain detectable in renal failure patients long after they are metabolized in patients without kidney disease.

POSTOPERATIVE CONSIDERATIONS

Small infants who receive adult organs may have respiratory compromise after transplant and may require posttransplant ventilation for hours or days due to increased intra-abdominal pressure.

DOs and DON'Ts

✓ Do obtain an ECG in any patient presenting with elevated potassium.
⊗ Do not induce anesthesia without treating metabolic derangements, particularly with ECG abnormalities.

CONTROVERSIES

- Large volumes of normal saline can cause a metabolic acidosis.
- Vasoconstrictors can decrease renal perfusion.

SURGICAL CONCERNS

When vascular clamps are released, you may note hemodynamic changes. Hypotension is common and usually requires rapid volume infusion to treat.

FACTOID

About 70% of children with chronic kidney disease develop ESRD by age 20 years. Children with ESRD have a 10-year survival rate of about 80% and an age-specific mortality rate of about 30 times that seen in children without ESRD. The most common cause of death in these children is cardiovascular disease, followed by infection.

60 MORBID OBESITY

Tatiana Kubacki, MD

YOUR PATIENT

A 15-year-old adolescent male presents with a history of morbid obesity, fatty liver, and severe obstructive sleep apnea (OSA). He is on nocturnal continuous positive airway pressure (CPAP) at home and comes to the operating room for a laparoscopic adjustable gastric banding.

> Height 167 cm; weight 192 kg; body mass index (BMI) 68.8
> Sleep study: Severe obstructive sleep apnea
> Electrocardiogram and echocardiogram: Normal

PREOPERATIVE CONSIDERATIONS

Obesity is classified according to body mass index (BMI = weight in kilograms divided by square of the height in meters). Children and adolescents with BMI >95th percentile or BMI >30 are defined as obese. Those with BMI >99th percentile or BMI >35 are classified as morbidly obese. The rate of obesity among children and adolescents in the United States increased from 5% in the early 1980s to 17% in 2010.

A comprehensive preoperative evaluation is important, since a variety of comorbidities, such as type 2 diabetes mellitus, insulin resistance, hypertension, asthma, cardiac abnormalities, fatty liver, the metabolic syndrome, and depression, are found during childhood in obese individuals.

Obstructive sleep apnea and obesity hypoventilation syndrome are common among obese children and adolescents. The prevalence of OSA is ~55%, with up to 20% of these having moderate-to-severe OSA. The definite diagnosis of OSA is made by a sleep study. The results of a sleep study are reported as Apnea-Hypopnea Index and define the severity of OSA. Patients with moderate to severe OSA are at higher risk of developing pulmonary hypertension and require preoperative cardiac evaluation.

An obese patient with a history of snoring or a diagnosis of OSA may be difficult to ventilate by mask and may be more difficult to intubate. Although the incidence of difficult laryngoscopy in obese children is much lower than that in obese adults, 1.3% versus 15%, difficult intubation equipment should always be immediately available. Anesthetics and opioids may cause airway obstruction and a poor ventilatory response to hypoxemia and hypercapnia in obese patients.

Lower functional residual capacity, reduced chest wall compliance, lung derecruitment, and airway obstruction predispose patients to hypoxemia and rapid desaturation after induction of anesthesia.

Peripheral line placement is more challenging in these patients.

Morbidly obese patients are at increased risk for compression neurologic injuries. At particular risk are the sciatic and ulnar nerves and the brachial plexus.

Highly lipophilic drugs such as barbiturates, benzodiazepines, fentanyl, and sufentanil have an increased volume of distribution in obese children and adolescents.

ANESTHETIC MANAGEMENT

- Place your patient in the reverse Trendelenburg position.
- Build a ramp beneath the upper body and head and carefully pad all the pressure points.
- Preoxygenate with 100% oxygen and CPAP of 10 cm H_2O for at least 3 minutes prior to induction.
- Obtain noninvasive cuff pressures from the wrist or ankle if the upper arm does not allow a proper fit.
- Administer subcutaneous heparin for prophylaxis against deep venous thrombosis.
- Consider dexmedetomidine infusion to minimize opioid use for patients with OSA.
- Propofol and succinylcholine should be dosed according to total body weight.
- Nondepolarizing muscle relaxants and opioids should be dosed according to ideal body weight.
- Anesthetic agents with low blood-gas solubility, such as desflurane and sevoflurane, facilitate faster emergence from anesthesia.
- Administer medications for prophylaxis of postoperative nausea and vomiting such as dexamethasone, ondansetron, or metoclopramide.
- Patients should be ventilated with positive end-expiratory pressure and a tidal volume of 12-15 mL/kg based on ideal body weight.

POSTOPERATIVE CONSIDERATIONS

- A semirecumbent position would help to prevent hypoxemia and atelectasis. For patients with OSA, nasal CPAP should be considered during the recovery period.
- During the first 3 days after surgery, the danger of life-threatening apnea in OSA patients is increased. Opioids and central depressant

drugs should be used with caution. Patient-controlled analgesia should be based on ideal body weight.

- Patients with severe OSA or significant cardiopulmonary problems may require intensive care unit monitoring.

DOs and DON'Ts

✓   Do prepare difficult airway equipment.
⊗   Do not give preoperative sedation.
⊗   Do not use isoflurane.
✓   Do rapid-sequence induction for obese patients with gastro-esophageal reflux disease (GERD).

CONTROVERSIES

Rapid-sequence induction for "airway protection" vs regular induction. Obese children without symptoms of GERD are most likely not at risk for aspiration, but there is a concern that they may have increased abdominal pressure in the supine position.

SURGICAL CONCERNS

The pneumoperitoneum can displace the diaphragm cephalad, causing the endotracheal tube to enter a bronchus. Absorption of insufflated CO_2 can worsen hypercarbia.

FACTOID

Research clearly shows that obesity has a negative impact on quality of life for adolescents. Teens with obesity are more likely to be socially marginalized then their normal-weight peers. Being overweight as a young adult can have a lasting impact on life satisfaction and aspiration. Several studies suggest significant improvement in emotional health and quality of life after weight reduction surgery.

61 MITOCHONDRIAL DISEASES

Teeda Pinyavat, MD

YOUR PATIENT

A 2-year-old female with a history of failure to thrive, hypotonia, and seizures is scheduled for a muscle biopsy for suspected mitochondrial disease. Her serum chemistries, creatine kinase (CK), and lactate level are normal. There is no family history of myopathy or adverse reactions to anesthesia.

PREOPERATIVE CONSIDERATIONS

Hypotonic patients should be carefully evaluated for respiratory insufficiency, cardiomyopathy, conduction defects, and difficulty swallowing. They may be at increased risk of aspiration, airway complications, and difficult intubation. Echocardiogram, electrocardiogram, chest x-ray, and serum chemistries are often evaluated preoperatively.

Anesthetizing the child with hypotonia of unknown etiology is problematic due to the unknown risk of malignant hyperthermia (MH), anesthesia-induced rhabdomyolysis (AIR), and lactic acidosis. Patients at higher risk for each complication are listed here:

MH: RYR1 mutations (King-Denborough syndrome, central core disease, mini-multicore disease with RYR1)
AIR: Duchenne's and Becker's muscular dystrophy
Lactic acidosis: Mitochondrial myopathy

Although the causes of hypotonia are diverse, and most are due to a central cause rather than to myopathy, clues to one of the previously named diagnoses should be actively sought by history and consultation with the primary pediatrician, neurologist, and geneticist. A positive family history of myopathy and elevated CK may point to muscular dystrophy or myopathy with RYR1 mutation. In these patients, volatile anesthetics should be avoided. Multiple organ involvement, especially of the central nervous system, and metabolic disturbances such as hypoglycemia and elevated lactate may point to a mitochondrial disorder.

Mitochondrial diseases are genotypically and phenotypically diverse and usually affect organs of high energy utilization (brain, skeletal muscles, kidneys, and liver). Common lab abnormalities include elevated pre- and postprandial lactate and hypoglycemia. MRI can show lytic lesions in the basal ganglia and thalamus. These patients are at risk of metabolic decompensation, including lactic acidosis and encephalopathy with preoperative fasting, perioperative stress, and pain.

ANESTHETIC MANAGEMENT

- Avoid prolonged fasting. IV fluids should contain dextrose.
- Lactated Ringer's solution should be avoided. Conversion of lactate to bicarbonate (a process that requires oxidative phosphorylation) may be impaired in patients with mitochondrial myopathy.
- Premedication is helpful in decreasing stress if an awake IV or IV placement with 50% nitrous oxide is planned. The patient should be carefully monitored for respiratory depression.
- Volatile anesthetics are not contraindicated in patients with mitochondrial myopathy, although some patients may be more sensitive to them. A mask induction with nitrous oxide and sevoflurane can be used.
- Other commonly used agents for induction and maintenance include dexmedetomidine, ketamine, remifentanil, and midazolam.
- As the muscle biopsy typically takes 30 minutes or less, the airway may not need to be instrumented. Mask, laryngeal mask airway, or intubation may be chosen depending on the patient's respiratory status and risk for aspiration.
- Careful padding of pressure points and patient positioning are essential, as a subclinical neuropathy may be present.
- Monitor temperature closely and keep the patient warm using a forced-air warming device.
- Increased sensitivity to muscle relaxants has been noted in patients with myopathy. If necessary, nondepolarizing muscle relaxants should be titrated carefully using a twitch monitor.
- A regional block may decrease requirements for inhaled or intravenous anesthetics as well as optimize control of postoperative pain. If the quadriceps muscle is biopsied, a femoral nerve block and lateral femoral cutaneous nerve block will provide adequate coverage.

POSTOPERATIVE CONSIDERATIONS

Hypotonic patients need to be carefully monitored postoperatively for respiratory depression and arrhythmias. Patients with mitochondrial disease should continue to receive dextrose containing fluids until intake by mouth is adequate, and postoperative glucose should be monitored. Pain should be treated using multimodal therapy, including a possible nerve block.

DOs and DON'Ts

✓ Do allow liberal intake of clear fluids up to 2 hours before the procedure.
✓ Do place an IV and start dextrose-containing fluid if the patient is required to fast for a prolonged period of time.
✓ Do attempt to schedule the patient as the first case.
⊗ Do not use lactated Ringer's solution.
⊗ Do not use succinylcholine as a first-line muscle relaxant. The administration of succinylcholine to a myopathic patient can lead to hyperkalemia due to the proliferation of extrajunctional receptors, or to MH if the patient has an unknown susceptibility.
⊗ Do not use a prolonged infusion of propofol. This may place the patient at risk of lactic acidosis and propofol infusion syndrome.
✓ Do treat pain aggressively and consider a regional nerve block.
✓ Do consider checking pre- and postprocedure glucose levels.
✓ Do try to use short-acting agents and monitor the patient closely for postoperative respiratory depression.

CONTROVERSIES

Although previously reported as being at higher risk of MH, patients with mitochondrial myopathy are now regarded as having the same risk of MH as the general population. Practice has shifted from avoiding volatile inhalational anesthetics to avoiding propofol infusion. Propofol as a single bolus should be well tolerated, but its safe use in patients with mitochondrial disease is controversial. It is postulated that patients who develop propofol infusion syndrome may have an underlying mitochondrial disorder.

SURGICAL CONCERNS

The muscle biopsy site is important. The biopsy should be taken from a site of weakness, but if the muscle is very weak, it may show only end-stage changes. The quadriceps is a common site chosen if the weakness is global.

Many commonly used anesthetics, including volatiles, morphine, and local anesthetics, although probably safe to use in patients with mitochondrial disease, depress mitochondrial function in the muscle biopsy specimen and may confound its diagnostic utility.

FACTOID

The ocular muscles are spared in many myopathies, but are affected in mitochondrial myopathy, myotonic dystrophy, and congenital myopathies.

62 DIABETES MELLITUS

Manon Haché, MD

YOUR PATIENT

A 7-year-old female with diabetes mellitus (DM) type 1 is booked for an emergency exploratory laparotomy for small bowel obstruction. She has been vomiting for 2 days, and complains of severe abdominal pain. Her diabetes is controlled via a continuous subcutaneous insulin pump. She also has a history of celiac disease and depression. Glucose: 210.

PREOPERATIVE CONSIDERATIONS

Patients suffering from type I DM have an absolute absence of insulin production and require an outside source of insulin to control blood glucose. This can be achieved with short-, intermediate-, or long-acting insulin preparations. Patients or parents should be able to inform you as to how much insulin the patient requires and what the correction factor is (how much insulin is required to decrease the blood glucose by 50 mg/dL).

Patients with type I DM are at risk for hyperglycemia and diabetic ketoacidosis, particularly during times of stress and illness. Note that ketoacidosis may present with symptoms mimicking an acute abdomen. It is important to find out the amount of insulin that the patient requires on a daily basis. Diabetes mellitus has several important complications, including neuropathy (including gastroparesis), nephropathy, vascular disease, and retinopathy.

ANESTHETIC MANAGEMENT

- Continue the patient's maintenance insulin at the same rate. Patients with an insulin pump may keep the pump if possible, and adjustments will be made with IV insulin.
- If the pump is discontinued, the patient's maintenance rate should be given intravenously.
- Measure the blood glucose at least every hour and make adjustments as needed.
- Add dextrose to maintenance fluids while you are running insulin, unless the blood glucose is >200 mg/dL.

- If the patient does not have a pump, an infusion of regular insulin can be started at 0.05 U/kg/h with a maintenance solution of D5% dextrose (D5%) (with NaCl 0.9% or NaCl 0.45%). It is better to have an infusion than to give intermittent boluses of short-acting insulin to keep the blood glucose more constant.
- In patients managed with a split-mixed combination of fast-acting and intermediate- or long-acting insulin (NPH or ultralente) or insulin glargine (Lantus) who have already taken their morning or daily dose of insulin, remember that the duration of its effect may continue for up to 24 hours.
- Hypoglycemia is much worse than hyperglycemia, and blood glucose below 80 mg/dL should be treated with D50% (0.5-1 mL/kg).
- Hyperglycemia (>200 mg/dL) should be treated by administering regular insulin subcutaneously. To determine how much to give, it is useful to know the patient's correction factor (= 1500/daily insulin dose). One unit of regular insulin will lower blood glucose by correction factor mg/dL.
- Patients with symptoms of gastroparesis should have a rapid-sequence induction (RSI); in this case, the patient's condition (small bowel obstruction) requires an RSI regardless of other considerations.

POSTOPERATIVE CONSIDERATIONS

Ensure that patients continue to be closely monitored until they are fully back to their baseline status. Continue infusions of D5% and insulin until patients are tolerating oral intake. Consult with endocrinology to discuss management in the postoperative period: if patients are to be admitted or kept on nothing by mouth for a prolonged period of time.

DOs and DON'Ts

✓ Do monitor blood glucose every hour.
✓ Do administer insulin and D5% with maintenance fluids.
✓ Do treat hypoglycemia aggressively.
✓ Do consult with endocrinologist.

CONTROVERSIES

There was a lot of interest in intensive insulin therapy and tight glucose control to reduce perioperative morbidity and mortality, especially in cardiac patients. This has now fallen out of favor because of multiple episodes of hypoglycemia encountered during attempts at maintaining tight glucose control (blood glucose 80-110 mg/dL).

FACTOID

There were no effective treatments for diabetes mellitus until 1921, when purified insulin was isolated by Canadians Frederick Banting and Charles Herbert Best.

PART 9

MUSCULOSKELETAL

63 HIP OSTEOTOMY

Susumu Ohkawa, MD

YOUR PATIENT

A 9-year-old boy with a history of developmental delay presents for bilateral hip osteotomies; he is bedridden and nonverbal.

Physical examination shows an undernourished male with bilateral hip dislocation.

PREOPERATIVE CONSIDERATIONS

There are many underlying conditions that cause developmental delay, the most frequent of which condition is premature birth. Prematurity may also be associated with other conditions, including chronic lung disease, hydrocephalus, intracranial hemorrhage, seizure disorder, feeding problems and malnutrition, history of necrotizing enterocolitis, gastroesophageal reflux, chronic or recurrent aspiration, and retinopathy of prematurity.

If the patient is taking seizure medication, it is important to maintain the medication schedule as much as possible, and to minimize any disruption of it. We need to evaluate the severity of gastroesophageal reflux. A history of central nervous system conditions, including the presence of a ventriculoperitoneal shunt, may be important if you are planning to use epidural anesthesia.

Evaluate the extent of respiratory reserve. Assess the extent of aspiration pneumonia or bronchodilator use.

ANESTHETIC MANAGEMENT

- Consider mask induction vs rapid-sequence induction.
- Malnourished patients are prone to be hypotensive right after induction. They may require fluid resuscitation or vasoactive agents.
- In patients with developmental delay, it may be harder to find a good endpoint for the extubation.
- Load epidural catheter with 0.5-1 ml/kg bupivacaine 0.25%.
- Maximal dose of bupivacaine (continous infusion + bolus) should be 0.4 mg/kg/h. You may add 1-2 mcg fentanyl to each ml of bupivacaine.

POSTOPERATIVE CONSIDERATIONS

Depending on the underlying conditions, the patient may need postoperative ventilator support and an intensive care unit bed. Use of epidural anesthesia with good analgesia may facilitate extubation after the surgery. The patient will usually get a spica cast. Create an opening in the cast so that the epidural insertion site can be examined if you plan to use epidural anesthesia postoperatively.

DOs and DON'Ts

✓   Do obtain a detailed history to evaluate the underlying conditions.
⊗   Do not interrupt seizure medication if the patient is on it.
✓   Do evaluate the risk and benefit of postoperative ventilation support.
⊗   Do not forget that most patients will get a spica cast after surgery.

CONTROVERSIES

- Placement of an epidural catheter can be confirmed using electrical stimulation, a radiopaque catheter, or water-soluble dye (Omnipaque 180, 3-5 ml).
- Postoperative ventilator use vs extubation at the end of surgery.
- Epidural use vs narcotics infusion postoperatively.

SURGICAL CONCERNS

A smaller femur head is at a higher risk for postoperative dislocation. Avascular necrosis of the femur head can occur.

FACTOID

Children in cultures where mothers swaddle children have a higher incidence of hip dysplasia. Swaddling brings the hip into forced adduction and promotes hip dislocation.

64 SHOULDER ARTHROSCOPY

Susumu Ohkawa, MD

YOUR PATIENT

A tall and thin 15-year-old male patient presents for an arthroscopic capsuloplasty of the right shoulder for instability.

PREOPERATIVE CONSIDERATIONS

There are anterior, posterior, and multidirectional instabilities, with anterior instability being the most common. Anterior instability happens to young male patients; the humeral head subluxates or dislocates anteriorly and can injure the axillary nerve, which presents as weakness of the deltoid and numbness of the lateral aspect of the shoulder. Atraumatic subluxation is usually multidirectional and is associated with connective tissue disorders like Ehlers-Danlos syndrome, Marfan syndrome, and the like.

An interscalene nerve block will provide superior postoperative pain control. However, the interscalene block is almost 100% associated with a phrenic nerve block, resulting in a paralysis of the ipsilateral hemidiaphragm. This can lead to respiratory failure in patients with marginal pulmonary function. Previous cardiac surgery may cause phrenic nerve injury, which makes careful history taking important.

ANESTHETIC MANAGEMENT

- For interscalene block using ultrasound or a nerve stimulator, 15-20 mL of local anesthetic are sufficient for adults. For children, adjust according to the child's size while following the recommended maximum local anesthetic doses. See Table 64-1 for recommended maximum doses of local anesthetics, Fig. 64-1 for the distribution of the block, and Fig. 64-2 for the ultrasound anatomy.
- Clonidine may prolong the local anesthesia effect. Add 1 µg/kg.
- Combine peripheral block with sedation or general anesthesia.

POSTOPERATIVE CONSIDERATIONS

The patient and his family should be given instructions on how to care for the anesthetized arm in order to avoid inadvertent trauma to the anesthetized arm.

TABLE 64-1	MAXIMUM RECOMMENDED DOSES OF LOCAL ANESTHETICS		
		Continuous Infusion (mg/kg/h)	
LA	Single Bolus Maximum Dose (mg/kg)	Neonates and Infants	Older Children
Ropivacaine	3	0.2	0.4
Bupivacaine	2.5-4	0.2	0.4
Levobupivacaine	2-4	0.2	0.4
Lidocaine	7 (10 with epinephrine)	Not recommended	
	3-5 (if IV regional anesthesia)		
2-Chloroprocaine	20	Not recommended	

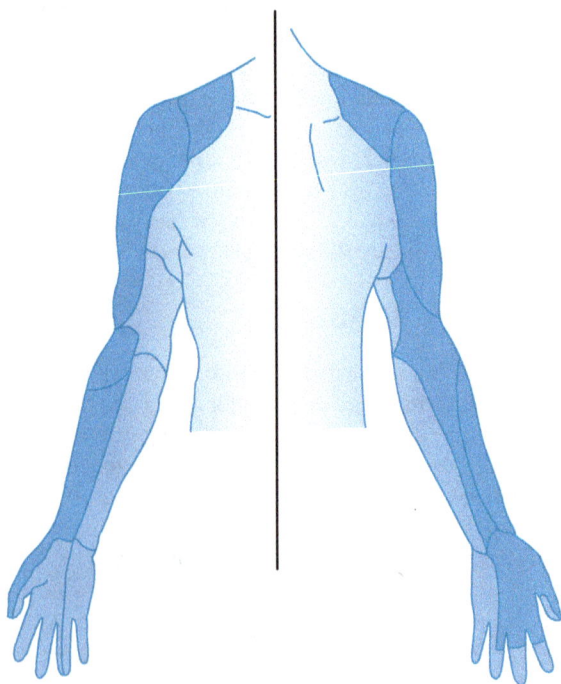

FIGURE 64-1 Interscalene block: distribution of blockade.

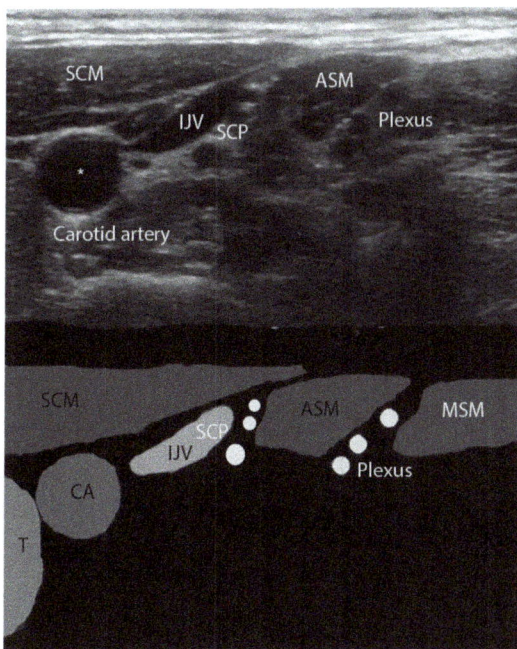

FIGURE 64-2 Ultrasound view of the interscalene area. [ASM, anterior scalene muscle; CA, carotid artery; IJV, internal jugular vein; MSM, middle scalene muscle; SCM, sternocleidomastoid muscle; SCP, superficial cervical plexus; T, thyroid gland.]

DOs and DON'Ts

✓ Do evaluate any possible underlying cardiac condition.
⊗ Do not hyperextend the joints of these patients.
✓ Do an interscalene block if appropriate.
✓ Use the shortest needle possible.
⊗ Do not do an interscalene block if the patient has respiratory compromise.

CONTROVERSIES

There is a case report of permanent spinal cord injury from an interscalene block that was placed while the patient was anesthetized. Some anesthesiologists perform this block only on awake patients for that reason.

SURGICAL CONCERNS

Postoperative physical therapy is an important part of surgical treatment.

65 CLUBFOOT

Susumu Ohkawa, MD

YOUR PATIENT

A 6-year-old child presents with a history of bilateral clubfoot. He has had previous nonsurgical treatment for clubfoot.

PREOPERATIVE CONSIDERATIONS

Congenital clubfoot may be associated with congenital syndromes, such as diastrophic dwarfism and spina bifida. Syndrome-associated clubfoot may be less responsive to manual correction and casting. Idiopathic clubfoot is often unilateral, but 1 in 4 patients have bilateral disease. Idiopathic clubfoot is very responsive to manual correction and casting. If a parent has clubfoot, the incidence in the offspring will increase.

The incidence of clubfoot is about 1 in 800-1000. It is usually treated with massage, manual correction, a series of casts, and percutaneous Achilles tendon lengthening (Ponseti method). This is effective in about 95% of patients. Surgical interventions including anterior tibial tendon transfer or foot bone wedge resection are considered for cases that are unresponsive to conservative treatment.

The procedure is elective surgery, and the patient should have taken nothing by mouth and be free from any acute illnesses.

ANESTHETIC MANAGEMENT

- Consider general anesthesia with mask induction and laryngeal mask anesthesia or endotracheal intubation.
- Use caudal epidural anesthesia or a combination of a popliteal nerve block and a saphenous nerve block. See coverage distribution in Fig. 65-1.
- The sciatic nerve bifurcates above the knee level into the common peroneal and tibial nerves. Both nerves can be blocked or block the sciatic nerve above the bifurcation (Figs. 65-2 and 65-3). The tibial nerve can be found right next to the popliteal artery at the knee crease. The common peroneal nerve runs laterally around the head of the fibula. Identify the two nerves at knee level and then trace up cephaladly to find the bifurcation level.
- The saphenous nerve is a branch of the femoral nerve. The nerve can be identified at mid-thigh, at the medial aspect of the thigh. At this

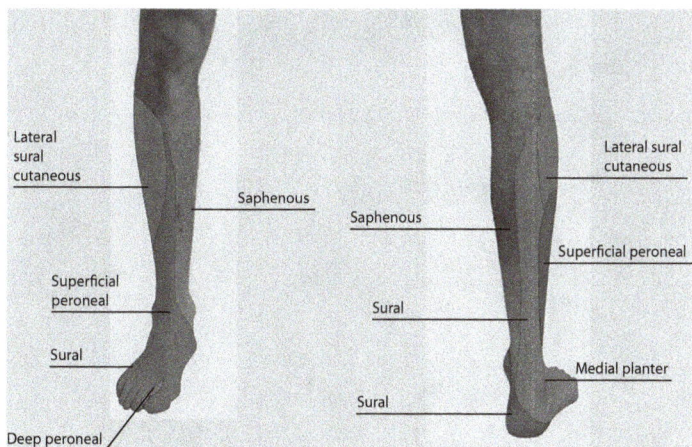

level, the saphenous nerve is right next to the femoral artery. The nerve can be traced distally from this level, and the nerve will be running right deeper than the sartorius muscle. At the knee level, the nerve will pass behind the insertion site of the sartorius muscle. Below the knee level, the saphenous nerve will be running right next to the saphenous vein, and local anesthetic can be deposited next to the saphenous vein.

- Use caution with muscle relaxants; if planning to use a nerve stimulator for a nerve block, avoid muscle relaxants or use succinylcholine and confirm the recovery using a nerve stimulator.
- Usually a tourniquet is used and blood loss is expected to be limited.
- Indications for popliteal block: Procedures on the lower leg, ankle, and foot (with or without saphenous nerve block surgery of the anteromedial aspect of the lower leg or the medial aspect of the ankle or foot) 15-20 mL

DOs and DON'Ts

✓ Do consider premedication with oral midazolam. These patients tend to come back for multiple surgeries.

⊗ Do not give muscle relaxants until finishing the nerve block if planning to use a nerve stimulator.

✓ Do use regional anesthesia. Use ultrasound to facilitate the localization of the sciatic nerve bifurcation.

⊗ Do not give narcotics to treat tourniquet pain.

✓ Do look for a meningomyelocele or arthrogryposis, since they are associated with clubfoot.

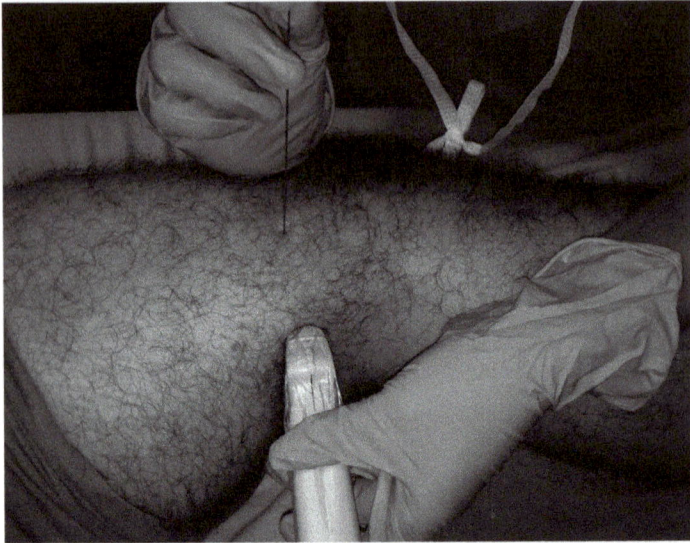

FIGURE 65-2 Probe position and needle insertion site for US-guided lateral approach. [The patient is in lateral decubitus, the side to be blocked up. The anesthesiologist stands on the side of the patella.]

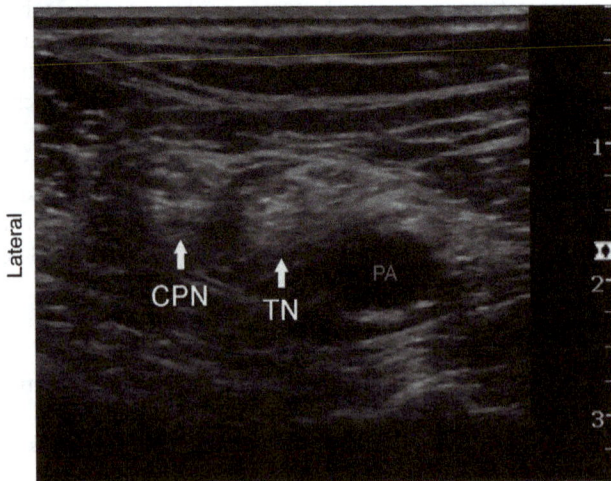

FIGURE 65-3 Common peroneal (CPN) and tibial nerve (TN) 3-cm above the popliteal crease. [PA, popliteal artery.] [Reproduced from Hadzic A. *Hadzic's Peripheral Nerve Blocks and Ultrasound-Guided Regional Anesthesia.* Figure 40-3b. Copyright 2012, The McGraw-Hill Companies, Inc. All rights reserved.]

of local anesthetic are sufficient for adults; decrease volume according to patient's weight.

CONTROVERSIES

Caudal epidural anesthesia vs peripheral nerve block.

SURGICAL CONCERNS

The talus is at risk for avascular necrosis. Overcorrection may result in disruption of interosseous ligaments. Correction may result in stiffness and restricted range of motion.

FACTOID

Kristy Yamaguchi, the Olympic gold medalist in figure skating, started skating as physical therapy for her clubfoot.

66 OSTEOGENESIS IMPERFECTA

Philipp J. Houck, MD

YOUR PATIENT

A 7-year-old boy with osteogenesis imperfecta presents with a femur fracture.

PREOPERATIVE CONSIDERATIONS

A mutation in the gene for collagen formation leads to bones that are prone to fractures. Different types of osteogenesis imperfecta exist; the severity ranges from mild disease to lethal. Patients have short statures, scoliosis, hearing loss, easy bruising, and hyperextensibility of joints. Type 1 osteogenesis imperfecta is associated with platelet dysfunction. Type II is the most severe form, with restrictive lung disease, underdeveloped lungs, and congestive heart failure. A cardiac workup is mandatory for patients with type II osteogenesis imperfecta.

ANESTHETIC MANAGEMENT

- Fractures can occur during positioning and during any manipulation, including airway management.
- Malignant hyperthermia is not clearly associated with osteogenesis imperfecta, but the patient can develop hyperthermia of unknown cause during general anesthesia. This usually responds to standard cooling measures.
- Patients often present with a short neck, kyphoscoliosis, and a fused cervical spine, which makes the airway management difficult. Basilar impression occurs when the cervical spine indents the skull.

POSTOPERATIVE CONSIDERATIONS

A delirious or agitated child may fracture more bones in the postoperative period; therefore, adequate analgesia is essential.

DOs and DON'Ts

✓ Be extremely careful with positioning the patient. If the patient is cooperative, find a comfortable position with the patient awake.

✓ Consider a fiberoptic intubation if a laryngoscopy is likely to cause fractures.

⊗ Avoid succinylcholine because fasciculations can cause fractures.

✓ Do start an arterial line in severely affected patients to prevent fractures from the blood pressure cuff.

CONTROVERSIES

There is one convincing case report of malignant hyperthermia in a patient with osteogenesis imperfecta, and there are multiple case reports of hyperthermia and metabolic acidosis that have responded to standard treatment. It is now widely accepted that malignant hyperthermia is not associated with osteogenesis imperfecta.

SURGICAL CONCERNS

Surgical options for patients with osteogenesis imperfecta include placement of intramedullary rods, surgery to manage basilar impression, and correction of scoliosis. The unstable bones make internal fixation very difficult.

FACTOID

Prince Ivan the Boneless lived in the ninth century in Denmark. He was carried into battle on a shield because he was unable to walk on his soft legs.

67 ARTHROGRYPOSIS

Susumu Ohkawa, MD

YOUR PATIENT

A 6-year-old boy with a history of arthrogryposis is presenting for an Achilles tendon release and tendon transfer.

Physical examination shows contracture of all four extremities, limited range of motion of the neck, and limited mouth opening.

PREOPERATIVE CONSIDERATIONS

Arthrogryposis is a nonprogressive congenital disorder. In most cases, it is not a genetic condition. However, genetic conditions may be found in about 30% of patients. Arthrogryposis is caused by fetal akinesia secondary to many different conditions (neurologic, muscular, or connective tissue abnormalities). Most frequently it affects the wrist, elbow, shoulder, hip, knee, and ankle joints, but in a severe form, all joints might be involved. This condition is not usually progressive, and physical therapy, occupational therapy, and surgical intervention may significantly improve the patient's quality of life.

Some arthrogryposis patients may have significant scoliosis and respiratory compromise because of restrictive lung disease. You may need to evaluate their respiratory reserve and create a plan for postoperative respiratory support. Significant involvement of cervical vertebrae and the temporomandibular joint may result in a difficult intubation. Careful physical examination and history taking are necessary for airway assessment.

ANESTHETIC MANAGEMENT

- Positioning may be very difficult. Good padding and protection of pressure points are crucial. Refrain from excess force during positioning.
- Consider awake intubation vs intubation after induction of anesthesia.
- Use caution with patients who have respiratory insufficiency.
- There are reports of significant postoperative hyperthermia. A trigger-free anesthetic may provide a less confusing picture when the patient develops hyperthermia postoperatively.
- Intravenous access may be very difficult to obtain.
- If the patient has significant respiratory issue, the use of regional anesthesia for postoperative pain control is recommended. Use a

popliteal nerve block combined with a saphenous nerve block or a caudal epidural block.

POSTOPERATIVE CONSIDERATIONS

Most patients can be extubated immediately, but some patients may need to be admitted to the intensive care unit for postoperative ventilation if they have significant restrictive pulmonary disease.

DOs and DON'Ts

✓   Do a detailed airway assessment and prepare for a possible difficult intubation.
⊗   Do not use excess force during positioning.
✓   Do use a trigger-free anesthetic to reduce confusion with malignant hyperthermia when patient develops hyperthermia postoperatively.
⊗   Do not assume that any hyperthermia is malignant hyperthermia.

CONTROVERSIES

There is an association with postoperative hyperthermia in these patients. However, there is no proven connection between arthrogryposis and malignant hyperthermia.

FACTOID

Positive end-expiratory pressure does not improve the restrictive pulmonary disease that is sometimes seen with severe cases of arthrogryposis.

PART 10

SYNDROMES

68 DOWN SYNDROME

Tatiana Kubacki, MD, and Manon Haché, MD

YOUR PATIENT

A 2-year-old patient with Down syndrome, who has had an atrioventricular canal repair and a pull-through procedure for Hirschsprung's disease, presents with a recent diagnosis of acute lymphoblastic leukemia. The patient is scheduled for lumbar puncture with chemotherapy, bone marrow aspiration and biopsy, and flexible bronchoscopy. The patient has been having fevers, has a chronic cough, and has multiple pulmonary nodules on chest CT.

> *Physical examination*: Anxious patient with facial features typical for Down syndrome.
> *Echocardiogram*: Normal cardiac anatomy and function.

PREOPERATIVE CONSIDERATIONS

Down syndrome (trisomy 21) is the most widely recognized chromosomal abnormality, with an incidence of about 1 in 700 live births. Airway management can be difficult as a result of macroglossia, macrognathia, and a narrow hypopharynx. Macroglossia and pharyngeal muscle hypotonia tend to cause upper airway obstruction. The nares and the trachea may be smaller than in normal children. There is also an increased incidence of subglottic stenosis. Disordered breathing during sleep, including upper airway obstruction and obstructive sleep apnea, is seen in 30%-60% of children with Down syndrome. These patients are at risk for congenital cardiac disease (mostly endocardial cushion defects, but also mitral valve abnormalities recognized at a later age). Pulmonary hypertension can result from cardiac disease or chronic obstructive sleep apnea. Patients with Down syndrome have an increased incidence of duodenal atresia, Hirschsprung's disease, hypothyroidism, and leukemia. They are also at increased risk for atlantoaxial instability. The American Academy of Pediatrics recommends getting an anteroposterior/lateral x-ray of the neck once between the ages of 3 and 5 years old. One should inquire about it, but it is not required prior to the patient's receiving general anesthesia. It is not a perfect screening tool, and we should always consider these patients at risk and use precautions when manipulating their cervical spines. To screen for pain or abnormal movement in an uncooperative patient, you can use keys, a light, a toy, or something else interesting that they will want to follow with their eyes and move it around them. Also, parents may describe regression in certain milestones, even regression in toilet training, or less tolerance for walking. These kinds of symptoms should prompt a neurologic evaluation. Ensure that you have a recent cardiovascular evaluation, and evaluate for any residual defects or pulmonary hypertension.

Remember that the degree of intellectual impairment varies widely in patients with trisomy 21.

ANESTHETIC MANAGEMENT

- Expect obstruction or difficult mask ventilation because of a small mouth, large tongue, and large tonsils, but intubation is generally easy.
- Consider moderate continuous positive airway pressure with jaw thrust during mask induction to prevent pharyngeal airway collapse.
- Avoid manipulating the cervical spine during direct laryngoscopy.
- These patients can present with profound bradycardia upon induction with sevoflurane, presumably because of a predominant parasympathetic response or abnormal sympathetic response. They sometimes do not respond to atropine; early use of epinephrine is recommended in cases of resistant bradycardia.
- Avoid muscle relaxants if possible, as these children are already hypotonic.
- A smaller than expected endotracheal tube may be required.
- IV placement may be difficult, and uncooperative teenagers may require a mask induction or intramuscular ketamine induction, even if that is not your first choice.

POSTOPERATIVE CONSIDERATIONS

Ensure that the patient's respiratory status is back to baseline. Any patients with preexisting sleep apnea or obstruction should be admitted overnight and observed with pulse oximetry. They may be more sensitive to opioids, so titration is key.

DOs and DON'Ts

✓ Do support mask ventilation with an oral airway as needed.
✓ Do treat bradycardia upon induction early.
⊗ Do not extend the cervical spine.
✓ Do use a smaller endotracheal tube as needed; check for a leak.
✓ Do inquire about recent cardiac evaluation and the presence of obstructive symptoms.

CONTROVERSIES

Many centers used to require a preoperative flexion/extension cervical spine film prior to administering anesthesia. Most people now agree that this is excessive and is not a great predictor for risk of dislocation in asymptomatic patients.

FACTOID

A simian crease is a single palmar crease, as compared to the two creases of a normal palm. This finding is frequently associated with Down syndrome. However, simian creases may be found as normal variants in 1 out of 30 non-Down syndrome patients.

69 DIGEORGE SYNDROME

Manon Haché, MD

YOUR PATIENT

A 5-year-old boy with a history of microdeletion of 22q11.2 presents for pharyngoplasty to treat velopharyngeal insufficiency. He has had surgery to correct a cleft palate in the past, and had tetralogy of Fallot, which was repaired. He has small pulmonary arteries and has had a stent placed in the left pulmonary artery. He also has developmental delay and chronic nasal congestion and cough. His medications include a nasal allergy spray, montelukast sodium, and albuterol inhalers.

PREOPERATIVE CONSIDERATIONS

Patients with microdeletion of 22q11.2, a segment of chromosome 22, will present with different phenotypes, and these may include syndromes previously described as DiGeorge syndrome, velocardiofacial syndrome, or CATCH-22. They may present with hypocalcemia in the neonatal period, potentially with seizures. They have a compromised immune system and are susceptible to fungal and viral infections. They often have conotruncal cardiac defects (truncus arteriosus, tetralogy of Fallot, or arch anomalies). Our patient had had a tetralogy of Fallot repair, but the extent of his residual disease should be evaluated. Specifically, on echocardiography, we want to look for a residual gradient across the right ventricle outflow tract, any pulmonary valve anomalies, and signs of pulmonary hypertension.

ANESTHETIC MANAGEMENT

- Micrognathia and retrognathia may make laryngoscopy and endotracheal intubation difficult.
- Careful aseptic technique is required, as these patients are at increased risk of infection.
- Calcium levels should be checked, specifically in the neonatal period.
- Blood products should be irradiated to avoid graft-versus-host reaction.
- Ensure that the patient is fully awake before extubation. Sometimes surgery is performed in a slight Trendelenburg position, and this may make airway swelling worse. There is a potential for airway obstruction postextubation, and using an oral airway may be inadvisable because of the risk of injuring the recent repair.

POSTOPERATIVE CONSIDERATIONS

Observe patients carefully to ensure that they are maintaining adequate airways, even during sleep. Ensure a return to baseline status and adequate oral intake before discharge.

DOs and DON'Ts

✓ Do ensure that you have a recent cardiac evaluation in patients with residual congenital cardiac disease.
✓ Do use a careful aseptic technique.
✓ Do be ready for a difficult intubation.
✓ Do check calcium levels.

CONTROVERSIES

Genetic counseling may be very difficult in light of the varying degrees of penetrance of this genetic abnormality.

FACTOID

Because of different phenotypes, it is now well known that DiGeorge syndrome, velocardiofacial syndrome, Shprintzen syndrome, Takao syndrome, and isolated conotruncal cardiac defects may all be forms of 22q11.2 deletion syndrome. This may be the second most common syndrome in children, after Down syndrome.

70 PIERRE ROBIN SEQUENCE

Gracie M. Almeida-Chen, MD, MPH

YOUR PATIENT

A 4-month-old male with Pierre Robin sequence presents for a tongue-lip adhesion procedure.

PREOPERATIVE CONSIDERATIONS

Pierre Robin sequence is characterized by retrognathia, glossoptosis (tongue falling to the back of the throat), cleft soft palate, and airway obstruction. With early mandibular hypoplasia in utero, the tongue is placed posteriorly, keeping the palatal shelves (which normally must grow over the tongue) from closing in the midline and causing a cleft. The rounded contour of the cleft differs from the usual inverted V shape of most palatal clefts. Pierre Robin sequence may occur as a component of many syndromes, such as Stickler syndrome, velocardiofacial syndrome, fetal alcohol syndrome, and bilateral hemifacial microsomia.

Neonates and infants with Pierre Robin sequence will have some degree of airway obstruction. Mild airway obstruction may require only lateral or prone positioning to relieve the obstruction. However, 25% of infants with Pierre Robin sequence have more severe obstruction, necessitating surgical intervention. Cor pulmonale can develop with severe chronic airway obstruction. Patients may also have vagal hyperactivity and brainstem dysfunction with periods of central apnea.

These patients often present with significant reflux and feeding difficulties secondary to anatomic abnormalities and with swallowing problems due to brainstem dysfunction.

The tongue-lip adhesion involves suturing the inferior portion of the tongue to the lower lip to prevent the tongue from falling to the back of the pharynx and causing obstruction. Once the mucosal flaps from the tongue and the lower lip are approximated, a temporary retention suture with a button is placed through the floor of the mouth and around the mandible to secure the repair. The goal of the tongue-lip adhesion is to relieve the airway obstruction and improve feeding until the mandible has had a chance to grow. The adhesion is left intact until the patient is approximately 1 year old, by which time the mandible has had time to grow and the adhesion can be taken down.

In infants with severe obstruction, mandibular distraction can be performed in infants less than 6 months old to rapidly distract the jaw.

234

Tracheostomy is a final option for the patients who fail conservative treatment, tongue-lip adhesion, and mandibular distraction. After the mandibles are distracted, the patient can be decannulated; it takes an average of 3 years for decannulation to occur.

ANESTHETIC MANAGEMENT

- Mask ventilation is difficult.
- Direct laryngoscopy and tracheal intubation may be extremely difficult or impossible secondary to severe mandibular hypoplasia.
- Consider awake, sedated, or anesthetized fiberoptic intubation, while maintaining spontaneous ventilation. Dexmedetomidine and/or ketamine may be titrated to produce the desired effect.
- When infants have significant difficulty with ventilation or intubation, aside from oral pharyngeal and nasal airways, a suture (0 silk) can be placed at the base of the tongue to displace the tongue anteriorly to assist with ventilation or intubation.
- Nasal intubation will be required for infants presenting for tongue-lip adhesion or mandibular distraction.
- If oral intubation is not desirable because of the nature of the surgery, tracheostomy may be required. Tracheostomy may be difficult if the patient has had a previous tracheostomy.

POSTOPERATIVE CONSIDERATIONS

The infant stays intubated postoperatively for several days to ensure the success of the adhesion. Extubation should be performed in the operating room when both the anesthesiologist and the pediatric otorhinolaryngologist can be present. When extubation fails, patients may require direct laryngoscopy, bronchoscopy, or tracheostomy.

Immediately after mandibular distraction, the airway may become even more challenging because once the distracters are in place, they may prevent effective mask ventilation.

DOs and DON'Ts

- ✓ Do maintain spontaneous respiration until the trachea has been intubated and lung ventilation confirmed.
- ⊗ Do not use muscle relaxants until the airway is secured and lung ventilation is confirmed.
- ✓ Do obtain a cardiology consultation if the patient has a history of obstructive sleep apnea and you are concerned about pulmonary hypertension.
- ✓ Do prepare for extubation in the operating room after a tongue-lip adhesion procedure with both the anesthesiologist and the pediatric otorhinolaryngologist present.

CONTROVERSIES

Optimal surgical intervention is not clear, and there is significant regional variation.

SURGICAL CONCERNS

Pierre Robin sequence patients may require multiple surgeries: ear, nose, and throat; orthodontic; and maxillofacial surgeries.

FACTOIDS

- This is referred to as a sequence rather than a syndrome because the small mandible and subsequent airway obstruction are secondary to a fixed fetal position in utero that inhibits mandibular growth.
- Although patients may appear extremely dysmorphic, intelligence is usually normal. When talking with patients, remember that they may have some hearing loss.
- Airway obstruction and difficulty of intubation usually improve with age.

71 TREACHER COLLINS SYNDROME

Gracie M. Almeida-Chen, MD, MPH

YOUR PATIENT

A 17-year-old male with Treacher Collins syndrome presents for mandibular and maxillary osteotomies.

Airway examination shows a Mallampati class 4 airway, large tongue, and free range of neck motion.

PREOPERATIVE CONSIDERATIONS

Treacher Collins syndrome is characterized by poorly developed supraorbital ridges, ophthalmic abnormalities, aplastic or hypoplastic zygomas, ear deformities, hearing loss, cleft lip or palate, macrostomia, malocclusion of the teeth, maxillary hypoplasia (narrowing of nasal passages, resulting in choanal stenosis or atresia), mandibular hypoplasia (tongue base is retropositioned, thereby obstructing oropharyngeal and hypopharyngeal spaces), and midface hypoplasia.

From birth, the adequacy of the airway is of primary concern. Repeated imaging may be needed prior to reconstructive procedures.

The degree of airway obstruction is related to the degree of maxillary and mandibular hypoplasia, choanal atresia, and glossoptosis. A narrow airway due to pharyngeal hypoplasia may cause respiratory distress and necessitate a tracheostomy. Tracheostomy may be required during infancy for those at highest risk for obstructive sleep apnea (OSA). Mandibular distraction procedures can be used to relieve airway obstruction and facilitate tracheal decannulation.

Limited oropharyngeal and hypopharyngeal space may lead to OSA, pulmonary hypertension, and in severe cases, cor pulmonale.

Aside from cleft lip and palate repair, the timing of the major reconstruction typically occurs during childhood or adolescence when the cranioorbital zygomatic bony development is nearly complete.

ANESTHETIC MANAGEMENT

- Give an antisialagogue for airway preparation.
- Mask ventilation is difficult.
- Direct laryngoscopy and tracheal intubation may be extremely difficult or impossible secondary to severe mandibular hypoplasia, a small mouth, and a narrow airway.

237

- Adequacy of mask ventilation should be determined. At this point, the airway can be visualized or managed with a variety of airway tools, with laryngeal mask anesthesia often being the only way to provide positive pressure ventilation prior to intubation.
- Use awake or sedated fiberoptic intubation if possible.
- Fiberoptic nasal intubation may be impossible due to choanal stenosis or atresia.
- If oral intubation is not desirable because of the nature of the surgery, tracheostomy may be required. Tracheostomy may be difficult if the patient has had a previous tracheostomy.
- Blood loss may be important during craniofacial reconstructive surgery and requires invasive monitoring of hemodynamic parameters (arterial line with or without a central venous pressure catheter), estimation of blood loss, arterial blood gas, and electrolyte analysis.
- Consider giving steroids to reduce airway swelling.
- Avoid excessive opioids to minimize risk of postoperative respiratory depression.

POSTOPERATIVE CONSIDERATIONS

Postoperative care often requires transfer of an intubated patient to the intensive care unit. In preparation for extubation, airway devices and staff support should be available in case the patient requires reintubation.

DOs and DON'Ts

✓ Be prepared. This is one of the most challenging airways because of the rare combination of difficult mask ventilation and difficult intubation.

✓ Do maintain spontaneous respiration until the trachea has been intubated and lung ventilation confirmed.

⊗ Do not use muscle relaxants until the airway is secured and lung ventilation is confirmed.

✓ Do order a type and screen and have blood products available.

✓ Do obtain a cardiology consultation if the patient has a history of OSA and you are concerned about pulmonary hypertension.

SURGICAL CONCERNS

Treacher Collins syndrome patients will require multiple surgeries: ophthalmology; ear, nose, and throat; orthodontic; and maxillofacial surgeries. Unfortunately, good cosmetic results are very difficult to achieve and do not last long.

FACTOID

Although patients may appear extremely dysmorphic, intelligence is usually normal. When talking with patients, remember that they may have some hearing loss.

72 KLIPPEL-FEIL SYNDROME

Gracie M. Almeida-Chen, MD, MPH

YOUR PATIENT

A 16-year-old female with Klippel-Feil syndrome on home biphasic positive airway pressure (BiPAP) presents for bilateral lower-extremity osteotomies.

Airway examination shows a Mallampati class 3 airway with a normal mouth opening, a reduced thyromental distance (3 cm), and inability to flex or extend the neck.

PREOPERATIVE CONSIDERATIONS

Klippel-Feil syndrome is the result of fusions of the cervical vertebrae such that the head appears to sit on the shoulders. The degree of severity is variable: type 1 patients have fusion of C2 and C3 with occipitalization of the atlas, type 2 patients have long fusion below C2 with an abnormal occipital-cervical junction, and type 3 patients have the presence of thoracic and lumbar spine anomalies in association with types 1 and 2. It is characterized by a short, possibly webbed neck, a low posterior hairline, and limited mobility of the cervical spine. Numerous associated abnormalities may be present, including atlantooccipital fusion, skull malformations, facial asymmetry, hearing loss, cleft lip, micrognathia, primary and permanent oligodontia, torticollis, malformed laryngeal cartilage with voice abnormalities, scoliosis, thoracic or lumbar vertebral anomalies, genitourinary abnormalities, Sprengel's deformity (wherein the scapulae ride high on the back), synkinesia, sacral agenesis, and cardiovascular abnormalities, specifically ventricular septal defect.

Patients with hypermobility of the upper cervical spine are at risk for neurological sequelae, such as paraplegia, hemiplegia, and cranial or cervical nerve palsies, whereas those with limited mobility in the lower cervical spine are more at risk for the development of degenerative disease. Syncope may be induced with sudden neck rotation.

Preoperative lateral flexion-extension radiographs of the cervical spine to identify patients with cervical spine instability should be considered.

ANESTHETIC MANAGEMENT

- An unstable cervical spine raises the possibility of neurological insult with head manipulation and positioning.
- Mask ventilation is difficult.
- Direct laryngoscopy and tracheal intubation may be extremely difficult or impossible owing to limited mobility of the cervical spine.
- A previous uncomplicated tracheal intubation does not assure repeated easy success, since cervical fusion is progressive.
- Adequacy of mask ventilation should be determined. At this point, the airway can be visualized or managed with a variety of airway adjuncts.
- Use awake intubation or sedated fiberoptic intubation, while maintaining spontaneous ventilation, using dexmedetomidine and/or ketamine.
- When patients have significant difficulty with ventilation or intubation, aside from oral, pharyngeal, and nasal airways, a suture (0 silk) can be placed at the base of the tongue to displace the tongue anteriorly to assist with ventilation or intubation.
- If oral intubation is not desirable because of the nature of the surgery, nasal intubation (which may be difficult because of narrow anterior nares) or tracheostomy may be required. Tracheostomy may be difficult if the patient has had a previous tracheostomy as a child.

POSTOPERATIVE CONSIDERATIONS

Extubation should be performed when the patient is fully awake and in the presence of protective airway reflexes.

If the patient is on BiPAP at home, consider placing the patient on BiPAP after extubation.

DOs and DON'Ts

- ✓ Do maintain spontaneous respiration until the trachea has been intubated and lung ventilation confirmed.
- ✓ Do maintain the neck in the neutral position.
- ⊗ Do not use muscle relaxants until the airway is secured and lung ventilation is confirmed.
- ✓ Do obtain a cardiology consultation if the patient has a history of obstructive sleep apnea and you are concerned about pulmonary hypertension.
- ✓ Do consider regional anesthesia as an adjunct to general anesthesia to minimize opioid requirements and expedite extubation.

SURGICAL CONCERNS

Maintaining the neck in neutral position is a challenge.

FACTOID

Klippel and Feil first described the syndrome in 1912 in patients with a triad of short neck, a low posterior hairline, and restricted motion of the neck due to fused cervical vertebrae.

73 CHARGE SYNDROME

Philipp J. Houck, MD

YOUR PATIENT

A 3-month-old infant with CHARGE syndrome presents for repair of choanal atresia. He has a systolic murmur.

PREOPERATIVE CONSIDERATIONS

All patients with choanal atresia need a thorough workup to detect other abnormalities of the CHARGE syndrome:

C: coloboma of the eye
H: heart disease (tetralogy of Fallot)
A: atresia of choanae
R: retarded growth or development
G: genital abnormalities (hypogonadism)
E: ear abnormalities (deafness)

Micrognathia may make endotracheal intubation difficult, and these patients are at increased risk for having laryngomalacia.

Choanal atresia can be membranous or bony, unilateral or bilateral. Bilateral posterior choanal atresia is associated with high mortality, particularly in patients with congenital heart disease and tracheoesophageal fistulas.

A small number of children require a tracheostomy to manage chronic airway obstruction. Severe gastroesophageal reflux and aspiration pneumonias may warrant a Nissen fundoplication. Swallowing and feeding problems may require insertion of a gastrostomy or jejunostomy tube.

ANESTHETIC MANAGEMENT

- Mask ventilation may be difficult because of the choanal atresia. Patients who snore heavily are at higher risk for airway obstruction after the induction of anesthesia.
- An oral intubation with an RAE endotracheal tube is usually preferred. The intubation may be difficult because some patients have micrognathia.
- Give dexamethasone 0.5 mg/kg, maximum 10 mg to decrease swelling of the airway.

- Patients should be extubated awake. Dexmedetomidine might be used for pain relief and sedation without compromising the patient's airway after the extubation.

POSTOPERATIVE CONSIDERATIONS

- Patients who have received stents should have a patent nasal passage immediately postoperatively; close monitoring is required.
- Patients with CHARGE syndrome are at increased risk for airway events after general anesthesia and should be watched closely. Neonates should be extubated in a controlled setting, most likely in the neonatal intensive care unit, with continuous positive airway pressure available if they have had significant airway obstruction, increased secretions, or aspiration.

DOs and DON'Ts

✓   Do have a formal cardiac evaluation for patients with choanal atresia.
✓   Do plan an anesthetic that results in a calm, spontaneously breathing with a patent airway after the procedure.
⊗   Do not be surprised by a difficult intubation and difficult mask ventilation.

CONTROVERSIES

Using stents for management of choanal atresia may not improve the outcome and can bring on stent-related complications.

SURGICAL CONCERNS

Restenosis in choanal atresia is an unsolved problem. No randomized controlled trials exist that show which surgical approach is most effective.

FACTOID

CHARGE syndrome was once thought to be an association, with no known genetic cause. In 1987, the underlying genetic cause was discovered (CHD7 mutation), and CHARGE association was renamed CHARGE syndrome.

74 CORNELIA DE LANGE SYNDROME

Radhika Dinavahi, MD

YOUR PATIENT

A 6-month-old infant with a history of Cornelia de Lange syndrome, seizures, and severe gastroesophageal reflux disease presents for a laparoscopic Nissen fundoplication.

> *Physical examination:* The patient is 3.5 kg and has short limbs, bushy fused eyebrows, long eyelashes, ptosis, and a depressed nasal bridge. A nasoduodenal tube is in place, and the patient has copious saliva in the mouth that she continuously spits up. On respiratory examination, there are mild rhonchi in the right lower lobe, and there is a systolic murmur throughout the precordium.
>
> *Medications:* Dilantin, Zantac, Colace suppositories.

PREOPERATIVE CONSIDERATIONS

Cornelia de Lange syndrome (also known as Brachmann-de lange syndrome) is a relatively rare syndrome. It is characterized by a distinct facial appearance, growth retardation, mental and psychomotor retardation, limb anomalies (short or missing limbs), bushy fused eyebrows, excessive body hair, vision and hearing abnormalities, gastroesophageal reflux, renal anomalies, seizures, and heart defects. These patients may also have behavioral problems, including self-stimulation, aggression, and autistic-like behavior.

Rhonchi in the right lower lobe may be the result of chronic aspiration due to gastroesophageal reflux disease. Consider a preoperative pulmonary toilet and/or bronchodilator therapy.

Patients with a murmur need a preoperative echocardiogram, given the association of Cornelia de Lange syndrome with cardiovascular lesions.

ANESTHETIC MANAGEMENT

- Careful airway assessment is essential to ensure that a rapid-sequence intubation is safe in this patient, who may have a challenging airway if the thyromental distance is noted to be limited. Carefully weigh the risk of aspiration against the risk of a rapid-sequence induction in this patient with a potentially difficult airway.

- Establish IV access in the preoperative area, and administer an antisialogogue to dry up oral secretions. Perform rapid-sequence intubation if it is deemed that the patient is not at risk for a difficult intubation. If the airway is challenging, consider awake laryngoscopy or performing a mask induction and maintaining spontaneous ventilation until the endotracheal tube (ETT) is secured by fiberoptic intubation, understanding that the risk of aspiration exists. Consider premedication with an H2 blocker and a prokinetic agent to decrease aspiration risks. Craniofacial dysostosis may make mask fitting difficult.
- These patients can have small airways, and you should be prepared with tubes ranging from far below what you would expect given the patient's age to the appropriate-sized ETT for intubation.

DOs and DON'Ts

✓ Do obtain a preoperative echocardiogram, as these patients have a high incidence of congenital heart disease.

⊗ Do not induce anesthesia without recognizing a potentially difficult airway.

CONTROVERSIES

The use of rapid-sequence intubation versus awake fiberoptic laryngoscopy given a possible difficult airway.

FACTOID

A diminished response to pain has been seen in some patients with Cornelia de Lange syndrome in addition to heat intolerance, so use narcotics cautiously.

75 EPIDERMOLYSIS BULLOSA

Philipp J. Houck, MD

YOUR PATIENT

An 8-year-old boy with epidermolysis bullosa (EB) presents for the insertion of a gastrostomy tube. He has a severe form of the disease and is completely wrapped in dressings. All his fingers and toes are fused, and his mouth opening is very limited. No veins are visible or palpable.

PREOPERATIVE CONSIDERATIONS

More than 20 different forms of epidermolysis bullosa exist, with different degrees of severity. All have in common that friction and shearing forces cause blistering, whereas pressure does not. Therefore, blood pressure cuffs are not problematic, but even a gentle chin lift can cause blistering. The blisters then form scars, which lead to deformity.

The scar formation after oral and pharyngeal blistering leads to limited mouth opening, dysphagia, and malnutrition. Esophageal scarring leads to dysmotility and gastroesophageal reflux. Scarring of the digits and toes causes pseudosyndactyly (mitten deformity). Anal fissures lead to chronic constipation. Chronic open wounds lead to anemia and to zinc, vitamin, and iron deficiency. Most patients suffer from chronic pain because of pressure in a new blister or infected skin.

ANESTHETIC MANAGEMENT

- Avoid prolonged mask ventilation to minimize the friction associated with handling the mask. Lubricate the mask.
- Laryngoscopy is safe as long as all equipment is lubricated.
- Prepare for a difficult intubation.
- Remove all adhesive parts from your electrocardiogram stickers and blood oxygen saturation probe. Ear clips or forehead sensors are useful in the absence of fingers and toes.
- Obtaining IV access can be difficult, particularly in a child that will blister from moving during cannulation. Consider premedication with midazolam and inhalation of nitrous oxide to facilitate IV placement. Inhalational induction in patients with an expected easy airway can cause less friction than starting an IV in an uncooperative child.

POSTOPERATIVE CONSIDERATIONS

Postoperative monitoring is just as difficult as intraoperative monitoring. A calm and pain-free child is the postoperative goal, since agitation will lead to movements that will lead to blistering.

DOs and DON'Ts

✓   Do insist on adequate monitoring.
✓   Do prepare for a difficult intubation.
⊗   Do not apply friction.
⊗   Do not slide the patient from the bed to the operating room table; lifting avoids friction.
✓   Do use a polyurethane foam dressing coated with silicone (Mepiform) instead of tape.
✓   Do listen to caregivers; they usually know exactly what causes blistering and what does not.

CONTROVERSIES

At some centers, bone marrow transplants are performed; their role is still controversial.

SURGICAL CONCERNS

Most surgical and dental management is as conservative as possible, because of the concern about blistering of the surgical site. The need for adequate nutrition with a gastrostomy tube needs to be weighed against the surgical and anesthetic risk.

FACTOID

The lay press has named the affected patients "butterfly children" because they are as fragile as butterflies.

76 KEARNS-SAYRE SYNDROME

Radhika Dinavahi, MD

YOUR PATIENT

A 10-year-old female child with Kearns-Sayre syndrome is to undergo surgery to relieve bilateral ptosis.

OVERVIEW AND PREOPERATIVE CONSIDERATIONS

Kearns-Sayre syndrome (KSS), also known as oculocraniosomatic neuromuscular disease, is a rare mitochondrial myopathy that is characterized by chronic progressive external ophthalmoplegia (CPEO), retinitis pigmentosa, and cardiac conduction abnormalities. CPEO affects the muscles that control eyelid movement and eye movement. As it progresses, these patients develop ptosis and ophthalmoplegia. Often, the muscles affected are initially unilateral, but the disease will ultimately affect patients bilaterally. Other comorbidities include cerebellar ataxia, proximal muscle weakness, deafness, diabetes, and other endocrine disorders. These patients typically have a normal early development until their preadolescent years, when the progressive neurologic issues surface.

It is critical to obtain an electrocardiogram to look for conduction delays and heart block. Cardiomyopathies have also been seen in older patients with KSS, so an echocardiogram may be helpful if symptoms warrant it. Family history may be helpful. The majority of cases of mitochondrial myopathies are not familial, but rather have an unclear pattern of inheritance. However, when cases occur across generations in a family, maternal transmission is much more frequent.

ANESTHETIC MANAGEMENT

- Always consider using local or regional anesthesia in these patients, if feasible, to avoid administering drugs systemically that may have adverse effects.
- Avoid prolonged periods of taking nothing by mouth, given that these patients are prone to lactic acidosis during times of stress. Try to schedule the case as the first case, if possible.
- Consider placing an IV prior to induction of anesthesia to avoid the use of a high-dose volatile agent for induction and its effects on cardiac conduction.

- Volatile agents have generally been used safely in patients with mitochondrial disorders.
- Propofol has been associated with profound acidosis in patients with mitochondrial diseases and should be avoided.
- Avoid lactated Ringer's for hydration, as it may increase lactic acidosis in these patients. Glucose-containing solutions have also been endorsed in patients with mitochondrial myopathy to prevent anaerobic metabolism and lactic acid production while taking nothing by mouth.
- If conduction defects exist, prepare an isoproterenol infusion and/or an external pacemaker prior to induction of anesthesia.
- Neuromuscular blockers have been shown to have no adverse sequelae in previous reports on KSS patients; however, given myopathy, it may be prudent to avoid them if they are not mandatory.

DOs and DON'Ts

✓ Do consider echocardiograms in patients with cardiac failure symptoms to evaluate for cardiomyopathy.
✓ Do avoid propofol and lactated Ringer's.
⊗ Don't forget to consider local anesthesia and peripheral nerve blocks.

CONTROVERSIES

Volatile anesthetics have been shown to inhibit the electron transport chain in vitro; however, they have been used successfully in patients with mitochondrial disorders for many years without event.

FACTOID

The mutation responsible for KSS occurs spontaneously the majority of the time; however, there are cases where it is inherited in an autosomal dominant, recessive, and mitochondrial pattern.

77 PHACE SYNDROME

Teeda Pinyavat, MD

YOUR PATIENT

A 6-month-old female infant with a large upper facial hemangioma presents for pulse-dye laser treatment. She is diagnosed with PHACE syndrome when workup reveals a small ventricular septal defect (VSD) and a right-sided aortic arch.

PREOPERATIVE CONSIDERATIONS

PHACE (or PHACES) syndrome is most commonly found in female, singleton, term, normal birth weight infants. It is diagnosed when a large facial hemangioma is associated with one or more of the congenital anomalies listed in the acronym:

P: Posterior fossa malformation. Dandy-Walker syndrome, cerebellar hypoplasia, hypoplasia of the corpus callosum, microcephaly, or absent pituitary.

H: Hemangioma. Large (>5 cm), segmental, extracutaneous hemangiomas on the head or neck; the most common site is subglottic, which may cause respiratory compromise.

A: Arterial anomalies of the head and neck. Abnormal cerebral arteries, saccular aneurysm, cerebral sinus malformation, dural arteriovenous malformation, Moyamoya disease, or acute arterial stroke.

C: Cardiac defect. Aortic coarctation and other aortic anomalies, patent ductus arteriosus, VSD, atrial septal defect, pulmonary stenosis, or cor triatriatum.

E: Eye abnormalities. Microphthalmos, optic nerve atrophy, coloboma, cataracts, third nerve palsy, or Horner's syndrome; unique to PHACE is "morning glory" retinal deformity.

S: Ventral defects. Sternal clefting or pit, or supraumbilical raphe.

Other associated findings may include micrognathia, congenital hypothyroidism, spina bifida, esophageal diverticulum, and sensorineural hearing loss.

The majority of children have neurologic sequelae—mostly developmental delay and seizures, and less commonly migraine headaches ipsilateral to the hemangioma, hypotonia, and central apnea. Routine evaluation consists of ophthalmologic exam, MRI or MRA of the head and neck, and cardiac evaluation including an echocardiogram.

251

Hemangiomas grow rapidly in the first year and typically regress spontaneously over the next few years. Treatment is required when there is airway compromise, visual impairment, skin necrosis, or infection.

ANESTHETIC MANAGEMENT

- Antiepileptics should be continued throughout the perioperative period.
- The IV line should be meticulously cleared of air bubbles in the presence of an intracardiac shunt.
- Careful airway examination for micrognathia is needed, as this may necessitate preparation for a difficult mask ventilation and/or intubation.
- If a subglottic hemangioma is suspected based on presentation or imaging, an ear, nose, and throat surgeon should be present for evaluation of the lesion and assistance with airway management.
- Mask induction and maintenance with a volatile anesthetic is normally safe.
- The airway can be managed with laryngeal mask anesthesia in older children, while endotracheal intubation may be more appropriate in infants.
- Maintenance of adequate cerebral perfusion pressure in the presence of abnormal cerebral vasculature is necessary.
- Use rectal acetaminophen at the start of the procedure.

POSTOPERATIVE CONSIDERATIONS

Postoperative pain is minimal and can usually be managed without narcotics. Prolonged apnea monitoring may be required for children with a history of hypotonia and apnea.

DOs and DON'Ts

✓ Do review the imaging of the cerebral vasculature and echocardiogram preoperatively.

⊗ Do not instrument the airway if a subglottic hemangioma is suspected.

✓ Do discuss the airway device and how it will be secured with the surgeon to maximize ease of treatment.

SURGICAL CONCERNS AND CONTROVERSIES

A flash lamp pulse-dye laser penetrates only 1.2 mm of skin and is indicated for ulcerated hemangiomas and residual telangiectasias that remain after natural involution. Laser treatment of an early lesion is controversial because of the potential promoting of ulceration and worsening of the later cosmetic outcome. Surgical excision is required for definitive hemangioma removal. However, it can be difficult to predict whether postsurgical scarring will be better than the results of natural involution.

FACTOID

Frontotemporal lesions are most commonly predictive of cerebrovascular abnormalities. Mandibular lesions are associated with subglottic hemangiomas.

PART 11

OFF-SITE ANESTHESIA

78 MRI FOR BRAIN TUMOR

Riva R. Ko, MD

YOUR PATIENT

A full-term, previously healthy 20-month-old girl presents for MRI of the brain with and without intravenous contrast. The patient has been experiencing progressive nausea, vomiting, and headaches over the past 4 months.

Laboratory: Blood urea nitrogen 22; creatinine 0.9
Physical examination: Patient appears somewhat lethargic.

PREPROCEDURE CONSIDERATIONS

Administering anesthesia in a remote location such as an MRI scanner is challenging because of patient inaccessibility, as well as the need for specialized MRI-compatible equipment. The scanner is always on. Absolutely *nothing* ferromagnetic is permitted inside the MRI scanner—this includes, but is not limited to, keys, pagers, phones, pens, needles, medication vials, stethoscopes, and oxygen tanks (unless specifically made out of MRI-compatible material). Credit cards and watch batteries can be ruined if taken inside the MRI. Many implants, such as pacemakers, aneurysm clips, and cochlear implants, are incompatible with MRI; if in doubt, it is best to check with the manufacturer. Gold and silver are okay, so most jewelry is not a problem. Many MRI centers will have a technician move a special wand over both patients and caregivers to ensure that there is no unknown source of ferromagnetic material. MRI imaging is not painful, but it does require the patient to remain absolutely still to obtain good-quality images. This is best accomplished with general anesthesia, using either general endotracheal anesthesia (GETA), a laryngeal mask airway (LMA), or propofol infusion and nasal cannula.

Because the patient has signs and symptoms of increased intracranial pressure (ICP), a rapid-sequence induction of anesthesia is indicated. Propofol and rocuronium are reasonable choices for induction agents. Oral premedication with midazolam may be helpful to prevent anxiety and facilitate IV placement, and to avoid possible further increases in ICP.

Make sure that there are no contraindications to the patient's receiving IV contrast, such as an allergy or severe renal failure, and plan to keep the patient well hydrated.

ANESTHETIC MANAGEMENT

- Use rapid-sequence intubation, and consider premedication with oral midazolam.
- Have a full general anesthesia setup both in the induction area and inside the MRI scanner. Use extra-long circuit tubing inside the scanner.
- Induction of anesthesia should be done in a separate induction area; transport the intubated patient with an Ambu bag to the MRI scanner.
- Opioids are unnecessary (this is not a painful procedure).
- Use MRI-compatible electrocardiogram leads, blood pressure cable, pulse oximeter, and temperature probe.
- Use earplugs for noise reduction.
- Maintain anesthesia with sevoflurane or propofol infusion with an MRI-compatible infusion pump; the usual start dose is 200 µg/kg/min.
- Keep the patient adequately hydrated; avoid increases in ICP.
- Monitor temperature carefully. Cover the patient in blankets and/or plastic as much as possible to prevent hypothermia. Hyperthermia can also arise because of the heat produced by the magnetic fields.

POSTPROCEDURE CONSIDERATIONS

Patients can be extubated either inside the scanner or back in the MRI induction area. Ideally, patients should be transferred to a postanesthesia care unit located near the MRI scanner.

DOs and DON'Ts

✓ Do use rapid-sequence induction or modified rapid-sequence induction because of the patient's recent vomiting and unknown ICP status.

⊗ Do not bring any metallic items inside the MRI scanner.

✓ Do make sure that full MRI-compatible American Society of Anesthesiologists monitoring equipment is available for use inside the MRI scanner.

✓ Do use an extra-long circuit inside the MRI scanner.

✓ Do keep the patient hydrated and covered.

⊗ Do not give ketamine.

CONTROVERSIES

- General anesthesia vs "moderate sedation"—who should be sedating pediatric patients for MRI?
- If general anesthesia, GETA vs LMA vs total intravenous anesthesia with nasal cannula.
- Role of dexmedetomidine?

FACTOID

In most parts of Europe, Latin America, Africa, and Asia, sedation of pediatric patients for MRI is performed exclusively by anesthesiologists; in the United States, Canada, Australia, and New Zealand, the majority of off-site pediatric sedations are performed by nonanesthesiologists (eg, pediatricians, intensivists, emergency room physicians, nurse practitioners, and so on).

79 CT SCAN FOR CRANIOSYNOSTOSIS

William S. Schechter

YOUR PATIENT

A 2-month-old infant with craniosynostoses is scheduled for a preoperative CT scan.

PREPROCEDURAL CONSIDERATIONS

Syndromes: This patient may have isolated, nonsyndromic craniosynostoses, or the craniosynostoses may be a component of one of the acrocephalosyndactyly syndromes (ACSs), which include:

Type 1 (Apert's)
Type 2 (Cruzon's)
Type 3 (Saethre-Chotzen's)
Type 4 (Waardenburg's)
Type 5 (Pfeiffer's)

Craniosynostosis is caused by premature closure of the cranial sutures and an associated growth arrest perpendicular to the involved suture line, resulting in a skull deformity that progresses over time until growth is completed. It is therefore important that this issue be surgically addressed early in infancy. It may be part of the previously noted syndromic paradigm, which is associated with brachydactyly (foreshortened extremities), syndactyly (fusion of the phalanges and obliteration of the natural web spaces), and polydactyly (extra digits). There is a great deal of overlap of phenotypic expression among these subtypes. Craniosynostosis may be caused by a new mutation or display either an autosomal dominant or recessive genetic pattern of inheritance. There is evidence of defects in fibroblast growth factor regions (FGFR) of the genome, resulting in abnormal bridging ossification of mesenchymal tissue.

Any suture may be involved (sagittal, coronal, or metopic), and in some cases more than one suture may be involved. Patients may be at risk of increased intracranial pressure: with one fused suture, there is a 15% risk; with more than one fused suture, the risk increases to approximately 35%.

Procedures include open strip craniectomy, endoscopic craniectomy, cranial vault remodeling, and spring-assisted cranioplasty.

ANESTHETIC MANAGEMENT

- For many of these young patients presenting for a CT scan, anesthesia is not required. The procedure itself is short and not uncomfortable. A brief period of sleep or nap deprivation, followed by feeding and swaddling just prior to the scan, will allow the patient to fall asleep naturally. The head may need to be taped in a neutral position, and several folded blankets may be placed against the side of the head to minimize movement.
- Anesthetic considerations for general anesthesia for a more extensive scan or surgical repair require a thorough evaluation of the upper airway, lower respiratory tract, and cardiovascular system are as follows:
  - Head size and shape. This will determine the proper positioning for assuring a good natural airway, proper mask ventilation, and optimal intubating conditions. Obtaining a sniffing position or a somewhat extended neck position may be a challenge if there is a prominent occiput or significant asymmetry. A neck roll or shoulder roll may be helpful. Patients with type 2 ACS have maxillary hypoplasia, which may cause difficulties with mask ventilation. Improvement in the mask seal may require choosing alternative mask sizes and mask cushion inflation pressure; occasionally, positioning the mask with the apex down can allow for a better seal. Nasopharyngeal hypoplasia and palatal anomalies must be assessed preoperatively and can complicate the placement of an oral or nasal airway or contraindicate the placement of a nasal endotracheal tube. Patency of the nares should be individually assessed, as should the relative size of the tongue in comparison to the size of the oropharynx.
  - Cervical spine anomalies. Flexibility of the cervical spine must be carefully evaluated. Flexibility or extensibility may be impaired.
  - Lower airway. Some syndromes are associated with anomalies of the tracheal cartilages. A smaller tube size than expected may be required. Neck and airway films may be helpful in selected cases.
  - A history of apnea or snoring should be obtained. This may foretell difficulties with obstruction during induction and may suggested the need for more intensive postanesthesia monitoring. Any infant less than 38 weeks postgestational age must be monitored for postanesthesia apnea until at least 50-60 weeks postconceptual age.
  - As a general principle, spontaneous ventilation should be maintained until the ability to ventilate the patient is assured.
  - Careful eye protection is necessary, since orbital size may be compromised and the globes may be prominent.
  - Often an inhalational induction can be carried out, followed by intravenous access. Choices then include:
    - For a brief scan, nasal cannula oxygen with side-stream carbon dioxide and an infusion of propofol (range approximately

25-200 µg/kg/min) can be used. If the airway is obstructed with spontaneous ventilation, an oral airway may be required.

- For a longer-duration scan or for intermittent obstruction during spontaneous breathing, a laryngeal mask airway (LMA) may be helpful. Anesthesia may be maintained with a volatile agent (sevoflurane) or a propofol infusion.
  - Surgical procedures or long-duration scans will require intubation.
- Standard American Society of Anesthesiologists monitoring should always be utilized. Since the patient is in a separate room (airway avoidance) during the scan, uninterrupted vigilance is required; often the patient can be monitored adequately through a window or by video. Apnea, dislodgement of an airway device or tube, laryngospasm, and aspiration are the major concerns.
- Since these patients have a high surface area to body weight ratio, temperature monitoring is essential.
- For surgical repair, good intravenous access is required; blood warmer and warm-air convection blankets should be utilized. Blood should be available for transfusion. Placement of an arterial line and an indwelling urinary catheter is advisable, especially if more than one suture line is involved or if the starting hematocrit is low (physiological nadir) at this age.
- Endoscopic techniques are being used with increasing frequency and are associated with less postoperative discomfort and less likelihood of significant blood loss.
- Venous air embolism may be an issue if the head is tilted up; trans-thoracic Doppler may be helpful in detecting this.

DOs and DON'Ts

✓   Do evaluate both upper and lower airway.
✓   Do have adjunctive airway equipment available (such as various masks, oral airways, LMAs, a videolaryngoscope, and a GlideScope).
✓   Do be aware that many patients with craniosynostoses are syndromic and may have significant airway atresias, clefts, vertebral anomalies, tracheoesophageal anomalies, elevated intracranial pressure, and genitourinary and cardiac anomalies.
⊗   Don't underestimate the risk of significant blood loss during traditional strip craniectomy or cranial vault remodeling.

FACTOID

Intentional human cranial deformation dates back 45,000 years to Neanderthal times. Hippocrates wrote of the practice of cranial modification of the Macrocephali peoples of the Mediterranean basin.

80 SPECT SCAN

William S. Schechter, MD, MS

YOUR PATIENT

A 13-year-old with refractory seizures presents for an interictal SPECT scan. The patient has frequent temporal lobe seizures that are refractory to intensive medical treatment. His current medications include levetiracetam, lamotrigine, and clonazepam. Planning for seizure surgery is commencing.

The physical examination reveals a thin, quiet young man with no appreciable disease. He appears afraid and tearful and resists lying down on the table.

PREOPERATIVE CONSIDERATIONS

Functional neuroimaging techniques utilizing isotopes are routinely used to identify a seizure focus.

When these techniques are coupled with proper electroencephalogram (EEG) analysis and MRI examination, a seizure focus can now be identified with high reliability and sensitivity that may allow for surgical extirpation of the focus.

The term *SPECT* refers to single-photon emission computed tomography. It is a nuclear medicine technique that maps blood flow. Since cerebral blood flow is usually greatest in areas of seizure activity, this allows us to identify an active seizure focus. In order to reliably do this, two scans often need to be done: an ictal SPECT scan and an interictal SPECT scan. An ictal SPECT scan requires the injection of tracer during a seizure. The seizure origination focus is identified by an increase in gamma emissions in the affected area. An interictal scan involves injection of tracer between seizures and is used as the baseline study for comparison. The tracer radiopharmaceutical usually contains radioactive technetium (Tc 99). The local tracer concentration peaks in the brain tissue about 2 minutes after injection, remains constant for about 2 hours, and degrades with a half-life of 6 hours. Ictal SPECT reveals both the onset zone and the propagation pathways. The ictal and interictal images are then compared to each other and to MRI and analyzed both visually and statistically, usually utilizing a parametric mapping technique in order to precisely delineate the onset zone.

Positron emission tomography (PET) scanning is a different technique. It utilizes fluoro-2-deoxy-D-glucose (FDG) scanning of the brain to assess regional blood glucose uptake and metabolism. A seizure focus usually displays *decreased* glucose uptake interictally compared to the contralateral side.

PET scanning is also commonly used for the identification of tumors, both within the central nervous system (CNS) and in the body as a whole.

Newer radioligand tracers are being developed to allow for the identification of specific neurotransmitters and receptor activation.

ANESTHETIC MANAGEMENT

Because of the patient's high level of anxiety, an anesthesia machine is brought to the scanner area, and an inhalational induction is performed with the mother present. The patient has a good natural airway. All American Society of Anesthesiologists monitors are placed, and an IV is started. A propofol infusion is initiated at 300 µg/kg/min and then reduced to 250 µg/kg/min. A second heparin lock is started, and the radionuclide is injected. The sevoflurane is discontinued, and a nasal cannula is applied with side-stream carbon dioxide monitoring. The patient, the infusion pump, and the monitors can be directly seen from a window outside the room. After 50 minutes, the scan is completed, and the patient is awakened and brought to the postanesthesia care unit.

Sedation needs vary depending upon the patient's age, physical status, and temperament. Young children under 6 or 7 years of age will usually require general anesthesia to prevent movement. Older cognitively approachable children often can hold still and may or may not require anxiolytics. Propofol, dexmedetomidine, pentobarbital, combinations of midazolam and fentanyl, and remifentanil infusions have all been used. Young infants may occasionally be swaddled with the arms at the sides. Restraints may be needed to prevent unwanted motion artifacts.

DOs and DON'Ts

For PET scans:

- ✓ Do have children fast for a minimum of 6 hours prior to the procedure. In addition to minimizing aspiration risk, this decreases endogenous insulin release, minimizing uptake of the ligand to other tissues.
- ✓ Do keep the room warm to prevent shivering and FDG uptake into brown fat. Avoid patient anxiety by utilizing the parents and child-life personnel. These two points are especially important for body PET (as opposed to CNS) scans and will improve resolution of the images.

✓ Do establish IV access in advance of the injection to allow anxiety to resolve.

✓ Do use normal saline, not lactated Ringer's, and do not infuse glucose for 4 to 6 hours before the procedure. This may require glucose monitoring.

✓ Do prevent otherwise needless repetitive scans and excessive radiation exposure by utilizing an appropriate level of anesthesia or sedation. Make the first scan work.

For both SPECT and PET scans:

✓ Don't inject through a central line (standard central venous line, port, Broviac, or Hickman). Residual tracer may remain on the catheter wall or within the reservoir. Some central lines cannot withstand the pressure if a power injector is used.

✓ Do use short-acting agents with predictable pharmacokinetics so that recovery will be rapid.

✓ Do be aware that inhalational induction of anesthesia off-site requires proper scavenging of waste gases. Consider an awake IV, if possible, and a total intravenous anesthetic technique.

✓ Do understand that waste products such as urine are radioactive. Diapers and secretions must be disposed of according to institutional radiation safety protocols. No pregnant caregivers should be in attendance.

CONTROVERSIES

- Often these scans take place at locations that are very distant from the main operating room and recovery areas. An institutional commitment to providing a dedicated nursing presence during induction and emergence is essential. Often these sites are so distant that more than one anesthesia provider may need to be present should an emergency arise.

- All of our agents affect cerebral metabolism and blood flow and may alter neuronal conduction and excitability. This may affect interpretation of the scan.

- Some radiation exposure is associated with the tomographic scan itself. Protect yourself primarily by ensuring distance form the source of radiation.

- Some nonanesthesiologists still utilize chloral hydrate for sedation despite the issues surrounding the metabolite ethylchlorvinyl's cardiac toxicity and propensity to create dysrhythmias as well as the environmental issues associated with the parent compound's disposal. It is favored by some for sedation of patients undergoing EEG because it does not depress seizure activity.

FACTOID

To their own psychological peril, anesthesiologists are experts at multi-tasking. In this universe, however, anesthesiologists do not exhibit the quantum property of *superposition*. That is, they simply cannot be in two places simultaneously. It is very difficult to remain "on call" for an ictal scan ad infinitum; all involved parties should agree on a rigid time frame in advance.

81 GAMMA KNIFE RADIOSURGERY

William S. Schechter, MD, MS

YOUR PATIENT

A 7-year-old female presents for Gamma Knife treatment of a right thalamic arteriovenous malformation.

PREOPERATIVE CONSIDERATIONS

The preoperative evaluation of such a patient is similar to that of any patient undergoing a procedural anesthetic. The parents should be made aware of the possible long duration of such a procedure and the potential risks of transporting a sedated or anesthetized individual from site to site.

Preparation for such a case is complicated by the need to prepare multiple non-operating room anesthetic sites, typically MRI (occasionally CT) and often neuroangiography for the planning stage as well as the Gamma Knife suite for treatment. Often there may be a significant delay between the planning and the actual treatment as the necessary calculations are made and reviewed. It is not unusual for such treatment to take several hours to the better part of a day.

This process must be scheduled and coordinated in advance so that there is minimal or no waiting time at each site.

Once it is in place, the stereotactic frame may obscure the airway, making mask ventilation or intubation impossible. The tools necessary to disassemble the frame must be with the patient at all times during planning, treatment, and transport to allow for ready access to the airway. For some frames partial disassembly to obtain emergency airway access or to optimize the head position for ventilation, will result in loss of coordinates and resimulation may be necessary. Some newer frames do allow partial airway access. You must be familiar with the specific frame being utilized, and staff members who are knowledgeable about its assembly and disassembly must be at the bedside. In an emergency, a laryngeal mask airway can sometimes be passed with the frame in place, and the patient can be ventilated through an attached flexible connector.

Since the patient will require MRI scanning, meticulous attention must be paid to avoid bringing ferrous materials or other non-MRI-compatible equipment such as oxygen tanks, monitors, leads, or probes into those restricted areas.

ANESTHETIC MANAGEMENT

- Local anesthesia in an awake patient, sedation, and general anesthesia, administered alone or in combination with local anesthesia, have all been utilized for this procedure.
  - For adults and cooperative older children or teenagers, anesthesia is not usually required. Midazolam is administered for anxiolysis (0.05-0.1 mg/kg), and an opioid such as fentanyl (0.25-1 µg/kg) is given incrementally. Local anesthesia (usually a 1:1 mixture of 2% lidocaine and 0.5% bupivacaine, not to exceed a toxic total dose) is injected at the pin sites where the stereotactic frame is applied.
  - In older patients a propofol infusion (approximately 25-75 micrograms/kg/min) may be utilized for sedation (monitored anesthesia care) or, alternatively a maintenance infusion of dexmedetomidine at a rate of 0.05-0.7 mcg/kg/h (boluses of dexmedetomidine are often avoided in young children because of the risk of bradycardia) may be utilized in patients who are cooperative.
- In general, it is our institutional preference to utilize general anesthesia with endotracheal intubation for patients in the pediatric age range (some carefully selected teenagers may be a rare exception). This is especially true for long procedures, highly anxious patients, and almost all young children. For safety, we prefer to do this electively. Our preferred technique involves oral midazolam as a premedication followed by an inhalational induction using sevoflurane in 70% nitrous and 30% oxygen followed by IV placement, preoxygenation, and endotracheal intubation. Induction is carried out in a designated anesthetizing location. Additional propofol is given as the pins are applied.
  - A propofol infusion or a propofol and remifentanil infusion is utilized for maintenance. Keep in mind that propofol exhibits a context-sensitive half-life and the rate of infusion will have to be decreased as the case proceeds. Propofol will also mitigate postprocedural nausea and vomiting. Muscle relaxation is not necessary, but many providers prefer utilizing it, especially during periods of transport and treatment. A bite block between the molars may be helpful to prevent tube occlusion in a lightly anesthetized patient.
- If angiography is performed, a groin puncture will be required. The patient must remain flat for 6 hours after catheter removal, and so an indwelling urinary catheter is always placed.
- Administer or monitor glucose, especially in young children if the period with nothing by mouth or the case duration has been long.
- A Jackson-Rees circuit is utilized to allow for spontaneous (or controlled) ventilation during transport. A full oxygen tank and portable suction are also necessary. A self-inflating ventilation bag is always carried as backup.

- Once in the Gamma Knife suite, the patient will be monitored by several videocameras. It is not possible for you to safely remain in the room with your patient because of the high levels of scattered radiation. One camera must be focused on the airway and another camera on the patient's chest, abdomen, anesthesia machine or ventilator, and monitors. You should be able to hear the pulse oximeter and see all relevant waveforms during treatment. You should able to assess for patient movement and proper ventilation. Emergency access to the suite can be obtained; an emergency radiation shutoff button should be identified during the preparation phase.
- Postoperative nausea and vomiting are prominent issues. This can be prevented with prophylactic ondansetron and avoidance of opioids for treatment of skull pain. If not contraindicated, ketorolac is often a good alternative. Steroids have synergistic value and are often requested by the neurosurgeon and radiation oncologist.
- Extubation usually occurs in the postanesthesia care unit or a designated anesthetizing area.

DOs and DON'Ts

✓   Do know your frame and have all tools and wrenches immediately available in a set location on the cart or stretcher that is known to all personnel.

⊗   Don't forget to remove all contraband prior to entering the MRI. The use of MRI-compatible monitors and equipment from the very start is advantageous. Make certain that oxygen tanks and transport stretchers are MRI-compatible.

✓   Do appreciate the value of an electively obtained, secure airway for safety and efficiency.

✓   Do monitor oxygen tank pressure and volume.

✓   Do carry extra equipment such as batteries for laryngoscopes and monitors; it can be a very long day.

✓   Do check the groin puncture site for hematoma or bleeding during the course of the day if angiography was performed.

CONTROVERSIES

- Depth of anesthesia needed: awake vs light, moderate, or deep sedation vs general anesthesia; airway device vs endotracheal tube; spontaneous ventilation vs controlled ventilation.
- Risks and benefits of muscle relaxation in an intubated patient who is traveling from site to site.

FACTOID

Non-operating room anesthesia for very ill children has become a fact of life. Although it was once dreaded, it is remarkable how experience, monitoring, sound institutional guidelines, and the notable, excellent help of nonanesthesiologists and nonsurgeons at outside locations have made what was once so onerous, safe and even routine.

PART 12

ADULTS WITH CONGENITAL DISEASES

82 ADULT WITH DOWN SYNDROME

Susan Y. Lei, MD

YOUR PATIENT

A 35-year-old female with Down syndrome and a history of a repaired ventricular septal defect presents for dental extraction and restorations. The patient has a history of obstructive sleep apnea.

Laboratory: Hematocrit 48%

Echocardiography: Mild right ventricular hypertrophy, mild to moderate pulmonary hypertension

Physical examination: 80 kg, 5 ft 1 in, Down facies, macroglossia, poor dentition, oxygen saturation 92% on room air

PREOPERATIVE CONSIDERATIONS

Down syndrome, also known as trisomy 21, is the most common chromosomal disorder found in the general population; it results from an extra copy of chromosome 21 and occurs in about 0.15% of live births. The risk increases with maternal age.

Patients with Down syndrome have characteristic features that are readily recognized, including microcephaly, mongoloid facies (flat face and oblique palpebral fissures), midface hypoplasia, and a simian crease. Hypotonia is another common clinical feature found in these patients, and this can affect the patency of their airways. When this is coupled with a narrow nasopharynx, macroglossia, laryngomalacia, short neck, and enlarged tonsils and adenoids, they are susceptible to chronic upper airway obstruction, leading to arterial hypoxemia and the development of pulmonary arterial hypertension. There is also an increased incidence of subglottic stenosis and tracheal stenosis because of complete tracheal rings.

These patients have varying degrees of mental retardation ranging from mild intellectual impairment to severe mental retardation. They tend to be very good babies, and as they get older, they tend to be content, cheery, good-natured and happy individuals with some degree of stubbornness.

Approximately 40% of children with Down syndrome have congenital heart disease, with the most common anomalies being endocardial cushion defects (50%), ventricular septal defects (25%), and atrial septal defects (10-15%). Perioperative mortality and morbidity for surgical cardiac correction are higher than for those without Down syndrome, which may be attributed to postoperative atelectasis and pneumonia, and preexisting pulmonary hypertension. Older patients with Down syndrome are at higher risk for having mitral valve insufficiency, even if they haven't had problems at a younger age. The presence of a murmur should be sought.

Atlantoaxial instability due to ligamentous laxity between the C1 atlas and C2 axis, resulting in excessive movement and subluxation, can lead to spinal cord compression. About 2% of patients will have cord compression, producing symptoms such as easy fatigability, difficulty walking, abnormal gait, decreased neck mobility, motor weakness, and sensory deficits. About 20% will have asymptomatic C1-C2 subluxation. The presence of atlantoaxial subluxation is readily diagnosed with lateral radiographs of the cervical spine in flexion, extension, and neutral positions. However, radiographic films of the cervical spine are not routinely done because the incidence of symptomatic atlantoaxial instability is rare, and these films are of "potential but unproven value" in detecting those at risk for spinal injury, according to a publication by the American Academy of Pediatrics in 1995.

Leukemia occurs in about 1% of these patients. They also have impaired immune systems and are susceptible to recurrent pulmonary infections.

The average life expectancy of patients with Down syndrome is around 50 years of age. This has increased over the last three decades as a result of improved healthcare and quality of life. Adults with Down syndrome are at higher risk for developing thyroid disease, eye disease, and hearing loss. They are also at increased risk for obesity as they age. Chronic arterial hypoxemia from airway obstruction and obesity can worsen any preexisting pulmonary hypertension, putting them at greater risk under anesthesia. By the fifth decade of life, about 25% of Down syndrome patients will develop clinical symptoms of dementia, and by the seventh decade, the prevalence increases to 75%. Almost all of them will display neuropathologic findings on autopsy identical to those found in Alzheimer's disease. They have a higher prevalence of mood changes, overactivity, auditory hallucinations, and disturbed sleep but less aggression than those without Down syndrome.

ANESTHETIC MANAGEMENT

- Consider premedication with oral midazolam; use this with caution if the patient has obstructive sleep apnea. Anticholinergic drugs may be needed to decrease oral secretions. Consider intramuscular ketamine for the uncooperative, apprehensive patient.
- Consider mask induction versus intravenous induction with 50% N_2O for IV placement.
- Obesity, hypotonia, and excessive skin folds can make intravenous cannulation difficult.

- Mask ventilation may be difficult because of the large tongue, flat face, short neck, and upper airway obstruction due to hypertrophied pharyngeal tissue and coexisting hypotonia.
- Downsize the endotracheal tube by half a size to a whole size for possible tracheal stenosis.
- Use manual in-line stabilization with the neck in neutral position and avoid extreme neck movements during tracheal intubation.
- Use arterial line monitoring if severe pulmonary hypertension exists.
- Atropine can cause overexaggerated mydriasis and tachycardia, but other studies have shown that these patients may not respond to atropine.
- More frequent and severe bradycardia with sevoflurane induction has been described.

POSTOPERATIVE CONSIDERATIONS

Patients should be extubated awake because of chronic upper airway obstruction and monitored carefully in the recovery room for postoperative apnea, airway obstruction, and stridor. Ensure adequate analgesia and antiemetic therapy because these patients may not be able to verbalize their discomfort.

DOs and DON'Ts

⊗ Do not hyperextend or hyperflex neck. Use gentle jaw thrust with minimal neck movement.
✓ Do maintain cervical neutral position at all times.
✓ Do use a smaller size endotracheal tube.
✓ Do take strict aseptic precautions during intravenous cannulation and central venous cannulation.
⊗ Do not give long-acting opioids until the patient is awake and strong enough to protect his or her own airway.
✓ Do explain to the patient what is going to happen in language appropriate to him or her, and consider having a parent or caretaker present for induction.

CONTROVERSIES

- Neck radiographs prior to surgery
- Atropine use

SURGICAL CONCERNS

Discuss with surgeons whether prophylactic antibiotics are necessary, given the impaired immune system of these patients, for procedures where antibiotics are usually not indicated. For dental and ear, nose, and throat procedures, the head may need to be hyperextended for visualization. It is important to communicate the importance of maintaining neck neutrality in these patients.

FACTOID

Since 1983, the Special Olympics has required all athletes with Down syndrome to obtain lateral neck radiographs prior to their participation, and those with radiographic evidence of atlantoaxial instability are banned from activities that are associated with higher risk for cervical injury. This requirement was supported by the American Academy of Pediatrics (AAP) in 1984. However, this support was rescinded by the AAP Committee on Sports Medicine and Fitness in 1995 because of uncertainty concerning whether radiographic evidence of instability correlated with catastrophic neck injury. However, the Special Olympics continues to uphold this requirement. In 2001, the AAP Committee on Genetics also issued a statement recommending that lateral neck radiographs be obtained between age 3 and age 5 years for Down syndrome patients. Most anesthesiologists will proceed with the surgery if the patient is asymptomatic and will take precautions to prevent excessive neck movements; those patients with neurologic symptoms will be sent for radiographic films.

83 CYSTIC FIBROSIS

Susan Y. Lei, MD

YOUR PATIENT

A 21-year-old female with cystic fibrosis presents for Broviac placement for total parenteral nutrition. She was hospitalized for a pulmonary infection last month, which has resolved. She also has pancreatic insufficiency. She is adamant that she should be completely asleep for the procedure.

> *Physical examination:* 35 kg. Thin female with intermittent cough; O_2 saturation 98% on room air.
>
> *Laboratory findings:* Hematocrit 35; international normalized ratio 1.2; prothrombin time 21; partial thromboplastin time 38; blood glucose 180.
>
> *Chest x-ray:* Flattening of costal margins, prominent bronchovascular markings, peribronchial cuffing, bibasilar atelectasis.

PREOPERATIVE CONSIDERATIONS

Cystic fibrosis (CF) is an autosomal recessive disorder that results from a gene mutation of the cystic fibrosis transmembrane regulator (CFTR) protein on chromosome 7. It is the most common fatal genetic disorder among Caucasians, but it can also be found in other ethnic groups. The identification of the CFTR gene in 1989 and substantial medical advancements have changed the once fatal childhood disease into a more chronic, progressive disease of adults, with the median survival age now being 38 years. Approximately 1000 new cases are diagnosed each year. It is estimated that there are about 30,000 patients with CF living in the United States, and about 45% of these are adults.

The CFTR protein is a chloride channel that regulates electrolyte and water movement across epithelial membranes. The mutation results in defective chloride ion transport with disturbances of sodium and water transport in epithelial cells that express this gene, notably those found in the lungs, pancreas, liver, gastrointestinal tract, and reproductive organs. Dehydrated, viscous secretions cause luminal obstruction and lead to destruction and scarring of exocrine glands. This results in pancreatic insufficiency, meconium ileus at birth, diabetes mellitus, obstructive hepatobiliary tract disease, and azoospermia. Mortality usually results from chronic pulmonary infection.

The gold standard for the diagnosis of CF is the sweat test. The presence of a chloride concentration higher than 60 mEq/L in sweat is a positive test in children. Clinical manifestations include cough, chronic purulent sputum production, and exertional dyspnea. Chronic parasinusitis is almost always present, and evidence of normal sinuses on x-ray is strong enough to rule out CF. Stasis of viscous mucus in the respiratory tract predisposes patients to *Pseudomonas aeruginosa* and *Staphylococcus aureus* infection. Recurrent infection and chronic inflammation eventually lead to bronchiectasis, chronic airway obstruction from mucus plugging, impaired gas exchange, pulmonary hypertension, and hemoptysis. Early effective management employing chest physiotherapy with postural drainage and mucolytics has improved these patients' quality of life and longevity. Those with poor lung function may require bilateral lung transplantation with a 5-year survival rate of 50%.

Blockage of pancreatic ducts will lead to the retention of digestive enzymes, which can result in autodigestion, destruction, and reactive fibrosis of the pancreas. Patients will eventually develop pancreatic insufficiency and malabsorption from impairment of exocrine and endocrine glands and will require enteral feeding.

If the patient has an active pulmonary infection, elective surgery should be delayed until the infection resolves and pulmonary function has returned to baseline or is optimized. Chest radiograph, pulmonary function testing (PFT), and arterial blood gas can provide important information concerning the severity and progression of pulmonary disease. Increased functional residual capacity, decreased FEV_1, decreased peak expiratory flow, and decreased vital capacity are common findings in PFT. Patients may have abnormal lab findings, such as hyponatremia, anemia, abnormal coagulation factors, and elevated blood glucose, that may need to be corrected prior to surgery. If cor pulmonale or pulmonary hypertension is suspected, patients will need a cardiac workup and echocardiogram to assess their cardiac function.

ANESTHETIC MANAGEMENT

- Monitored anesthesia care should be considered, but this may be difficult in an uncooperative patient. Administering higher doses of sedation may cause hypoventilation and decreased cough, which could worsen atelectasis and pulmonary hypertension.
- Intravenous induction is preferred. In a younger patient, mask induction is a good alternative, but induction may be prolonged as a result of pulmonary disease, and thick airway secretions can impede gas exchange and diffusion.
- In a case where this is an alternative, consider regional anesthesia to improve the chance for extubation. Prolonged intubation predisposes to pulmonary infection and barotrauma.

- Humidify and warm inspired gases to avoid drying of secretions.
- Frequent, aggressive suctioning of the airway is necessary, and intubation will facilitate pulmonary toilet.
- Intubate after the patient is deeply anesthestized and relaxed because coughing and laryngospasm are common as a result of airway hyperreactivity.
- Consider rapid-sequence induction because these patients are at high risk for gastroesophageal reflux and perioperative aspiration. Chronic coughing and lung hyperinflation resulting in a depressed diaphragm increase the intra-abdominal pressure and contribute to gastroesophageal reflux disease (GERD). About 50% of CF patients will have GERD by age 6.
- Maintain close glucose monitoring and administer insulin therapy as needed.
- Anesthesia can be maintained with sevoflurane or isoflurane, which can help decrease airway resistance and hyperactivity. Desflurane should be avoided because it can irritate the airway.
- Avoid high airway pressures during assisted or controlled ventilation, especially in the presence of bullae that can lead to pneumothorax.
- Bronchodilators such as beta-adrenergic agonists can decrease airway reactivity, but adults can develop worsening of expiratory airflow in response to the drug; this is attributed to progressive loss of airway cartilaginous support from chronic inflammation and fibrosis. This can further complicate airway obstruction.
- Use aggressive suctioning with normal saline lavage of the endotracheal tube prior to extubation, and extubate only after airway reflexes, especially the cough reflex, have fully recovered.
- Limit narcotic use to avoid hypoventilation after extubation.

POSTOPERATIVE CONSIDERATIONS

Cystic fibrosis patients are at high risk for recurrent pulmonary infections. Therefore, early extubation is of paramount importance because prolonged intubation and mechanical ventilation contributes significantly to the morbidity and mortality of these patients. Adequate postoperative pain management is critical to respiratory function, combined with adjuvant drugs to prevent respiratory depression and to encourage coughing, deep breathing, and mobilization of viscous secretions.

DOs and DON'Ts

✓ Do humidify inspired gases.
✓ Do consider regional anesthesia and adjuvants.
✓ Do give stress dose steroids if the patient has taken steroids for pulmonary exacerbation in the past year.

(continued)

✓   Do use caution with the use of respiratory depressants and
     sedatives.
⊗   Do not give ketamine, which can increase bronchial secretions.
⊗   Do not use nitrous oxide, which can rupture bullae and cause
     pneumothorax.
✓   Do use a cuffed endotracheal tube as these patients may have
     decreased lung compliance.
⊗   Do not give histamine-releasing drugs, ie, morphine or thiopental,
     as they can cause bronchial hyperactivity.
✓   Do plan for extubation at the end of the procedure to decrease
     morbidity and mortality.

CONTROVERSIES

Anticholinergic use: some believe that it can decrease the volume of
secretions but not thicken secretions, while others believe that it can dry
out secretions, further worsening airway obstruction. Its use remains
controversial.

SURGICAL CONCERNS

Pancreatic insufficiency can lead to malabsorption of vitamin K in the
gut, resulting in a deficiency of vitamin K-dependent coagulation factors, leading to a coagulopathy. It is important to send coagulation tests
preoperatively and treat with vitamin K before surgery if necessary.

FACTOID

The most common genetic defect of the CFTR gene is the ΔF08 mutation,
which is responsible for 90% of CF cases in the United States and accounts
for 70% of defective alleles. The mutation codes for an abnormal, misfolded
protein that is rapidly degraded before it reaches the cell membrane. However, there is tremendous variability in terms of clinical severity associated
with this mutation because of ethnic diversity among the American population. In addition, research has shown that the genotype does not correlate
with the phenotypic severity of the disease.

84 FONTAN PHYSIOLOGY

Susan Y. Lei, MD

YOUR PATIENT

A 25-year-old man with hypoplastic left heart syndrome who had a Fontan procedure 20 years ago presents for laparoscopic appendectomy. He complains of right lower quadrant pain for 2 days with nausea and vomiting, which has now resolved. He has had decreased oral intake because of the pain. An IV was started, and he was given 1 L of lactated Ringer's in the emergency room. He was also started on ampicillin/sulbactam and morphine in the emergency room.

Physical examination: 85-kg male, well developed.

Echocardiogram: Qualitatively good ventricular function, no intra-atrial shunting, patent Fontan pathways, trivial triscuspid regurgitation.

Labs: White blood count 18; hematocrit 41.

Ultrasound: Inflamed appendix.

PREOPERATIVE CONSIDERATIONS

Advancements in the medical and surgical management of complex congenital cardiac diseases requiring staged single ventricle procedures and ultimately palliated to Fontan physiology have improved survival into adulthood. More of these patients are now presenting for noncardiac surgery and pose a challenge to anesthesiologists who are not used to taking care of patients with congenital cardiac disease.

The first successful Fontan procedure was published by Norwood in 1983, and these patients have now reached adulthood. In Fontan physiology, systemic venous blood passively flows directly into the pulmonary circulation to be oxygenated and returns to a common atrium and single ventricle in the heart to perfuse the systemic circulation. The primary driving force promoting pulmonary blood flow and eventually cardiac output is the transpulmonary gradient, which is the difference between central venous pressure and systemic ventricular end-diastolic pressure. Factors that affect blood flow include systemic venous pressure and volume, pulmonary vascular resistance, cardiac rhythm, and ventricular function. Any perturbations in these factors can compromise blood flow and cardiac output.

It is necessary to inquire about feeding status, any episodes of vomiting and diarrhea, and decreased appetite to assess fluid status because there can be severe hypotension upon induction of anesthesia. It is important to maintain normovolemia prior to any anesthetic induction. Obtain an electrocardiogram and an echocardiogram to assess for ventricular function, intracardiac shunting, patency of the Fontan circuit, and valvular function. Prior catheterization reports may provide additional information about pressures in the Fontan circulation.

ANESTHETIC MANAGEMENT

- Give an intravenous fluid bolus prior to induction. This is even more important in patients who are to undergo laparoscopic procedures because insufflation of the abdomen will further decrease venous return and cardiac output.
- Place intermittent pneumatic compression device on legs prior to induction because blood flow is sluggish, so these patients are at risk for thromboembolic events.
- Avoid drugs that can cause myocardial depression or reduce ventricular function.
- Consider using midazolam, fentanyl, etomidate and rocuronium for induction of anesthesia.
- Consider maintenance with a narcotic-based anesthetic such as remifentanil infusion to maintain cardiac stability and to decrease minimum alveolar concentration requirements of anesthetic gas.
- Ask surgeons to keep insufflation pressures less than 12 cm H_2O.
- Ensure appropriate ventilation to maintain adequate lung volumes and gas exchange. Avoid excessive positive end-expiratory pressure (PEEP), which can increase intrathoracic pressures.
- Extubate at the end of surgery because positive pressure ventilation increases intrathoracic pressure, thereby decreasing venous return.

POSTOPERATIVE CONSIDERATIONS

Patients should be monitored closely in the recovery room for cardiac function. It is important to monitor fluid status, oral intake, and urine output to ensure that patients remain normovolemic. For major surgeries, they should be admitted to the intensive care unit postoperatively.

DOs and DON'Ts

- ✓ Do give a fluid bolus prior to induction.
- ✓ Do keep insufflation pressures less than 12 cm H_2O.
- ✓ Do plan for early extubation.
- ⊗ Do avoid ventilation with high peak airway pressures and PEEP.

CONTROVERSIES

Neuroaxial anesthetic techniques, especially spinal techniques, can lead to severe hypotension as a result of blockage of cardioaccelerator fibers in the spinal cord. On the ther hand, peripheral nerve blocks are associated with minimal cardiac instability.

SURGICAL CONCERNS

Patients who undergo laparoscopic appendectomy are usually placed in the Trendelenburg position to improve visualization of the surgical field. This positioning and CO_2 insufflation of the abdomen can increase intra-abdominal and intrathoracic pressures and increase the airway pressures needed to maintain adequate ventilation, which can compromise the Fontan physiology. Studies have shown that insufflation pressures of less than 12 cm H_2O did not decrease cardiac output, whereas pressures of more than 15-20 cm H_2O did. If the patient becomes hemodynamically unstable, discuss converting to an open procedure with the surgeon.

FACTOID

There have been reports of CO_2 emboli from insufflation pressures of 18-20 cm H_2O; this can severely limit pulmonary blood flow and cardiac output in Fontan patients, whose pulmonary flow is passive. The presence of a fenestrated Fontan circuit further puts them at risk for paradoxical CO_2 embolism to the coronary and cerebral circulations.

85 EISENMENGER SYNDROME

Susan Y. Lei, MD

YOUR PATIENT

A 30-year-old female with an unrepaired patent ductus arteriosus and Eisenmenger syndrome presents for laparoscopic ovarian cystectomy.

Electrocardiogram: Normal sinus rhythm at 75 bpm, right ventricular hypertrophy (RVH).

Echocardiogram: Moderately decreased right ventricular function, moderate RVH, bowing interventricular septum.

Physical examination: 65-kg female with 92% O_2 saturation on room air.

PREOPERATIVE CONSIDERATIONS

Eisenmenger syndrome occurs when a congenital cardiac defect with left-to-right shunting reverses direction as a result of marked elevations in pulmonary vascular resistance to a level equal to or exceeding systemic vascular resistance. The shunt becomes either bidirectional or right to left. Exposure of the pulmonary vasculature to increased blood flow and pressure, as seen frequently in intracardiac shunts, results in pulmonary obstructive disease. In the early stage, this is confined to the arteriolar musculature and is still amenable to pharmacological treatment or surgical correction. However, if the cardiac defect remains uncorrected, the pulmonary vasculature changes will become fixed, and surgical correction at this point carries a very high mortality rate. Shunt reversal occurs in 50% of unrepaired ventricular septal defects and 10% of unrepaired atrial septal defects.

Signs and symptoms include cyanosis, decreased exercise tolerance, palpitations from atrial fibrillation or atrial flutter, and arterial hypoxemia leading to erythrocytosis and polycythemia with visual disturbances, headache, dizziness, and paresthesias. Patients can present with hemoptysis from pulmonary infarction or rupture of dilated pulmonary vessels. There is an increased risk of cerebral vascular accidents or brain abscesses from paradoxical emboli. Both coagulopathy and thrombotic events can occur. The cardiac output becomes fixed as a result of fixed elevated pulmonary vascular resistance, and patients become preload dependent to maintain cardiac output. Syncopal episodes can occur when cardiac output is inadequate, and sudden death is possible.

Treatment with intravenous epoprostenol may be beneficial, but no treatment has been proven effective. Correction of the cardiac defect with concurrent lung transplantation or combined lung-heart transplantation is possible only for a select few. Symptoms of hyperviscosity may be relieved with phlebotomy with isovolemic replacement.

Patients with fixed pulmonary vascular resistance, by definition, will not respond to pharmacologic intervention, but some patients' pulmonary circulation may retain some degree of reactivity to pulmonary vasodilators such as nitric oxide or inhaled prostacyclin.

ANESTHETIC MANAGEMENT

- Maintain the preoperative level of systemic vascular resistance and avoid vasodilating drugs that can increase right-to-left shunting. Norepinephrine infusion can help maintain systemic vascular resistance. Epinephrine and vasopressin infusions may also be used.
- Maintain preload because cardiac output is fixed. If the patient is taking nothing by mouth for extended periods of time prior to the procedure, consider giving a fluid bolus before anesthetic induction.
- Remove all bubbles in IV lines.
- Consider prophylactic phlebotomy with isovolemic replacement if hematocrit is higher than 60%.
- Consider preinduction arterial monitoring and IV induction.
- Have nitric oxide in the operating room prior to induction.
- Use antibiotic prophylaxis as indicated.
- Maintain systemic arterial blood pressure to ensure adequate coronary perfusion of the hypertrophied right ventricle. Give phenylephrine boluses when necessary.
- Plan for early tracheal extubation because positive pressure ventilation increases pulmonary vascular resistance.
- Laparoscopy is not a good option in this patient, who will not tolerate the decrease in preload caused by increased intra-abdominal pressure or the potential hypercarbia caused by insufflating CO_2 and decreased lung compliance.

POSTOPERATIVE CONSIDERATIONS

Patients should be normovolemic in the postoperative period. Oral intake should resume as soon as possible. Pain control is critical to maintain adequate ventilation, but opioids should be given cautiously to avoid oversedation and hypoxia.

DOs and DON'Ts

- ✓ Do maintain systemic blood pressure and systemic vascular resistance.
- ✓ Do have vasoconstrictors, such as phenylephrine, readily available.
- ⊗ Do not use myocardial depressants, especially when there is right ventricular dysfunction.
- ⊗ Do not place a pulmonary artery catheter unless the benefits significantly outweigh the risks because there is a high risk of pulmonary artery rupture.

CONTROVERSIES

Regional anesthesia, which is normally accompanied by decreased systemic vascular resistance and systemic blood pressure, has been successful in some cases when drugs are given slowly with close monitoring of blood pressure and oxygen saturation. Avoid epinephrine in an epidural, as this has been associated with an exaggerated decrease in systemic vascular resistance because of its peripheral beta-agonist effects. Consider phenylephrine infusion to maintain systemic vascular resistance.

SURGICAL CONCERNS

Laparoscopic procedures can pose an increased risk because abdominal insufflation can increase the $PaCO_2$, resulting in acidosis, hypotension, and cardiac arrhythmias. Also, abdominal insufflation can cause a decrease in preload, which this patient may not tolerate. Ventilatory maneuvers to maintain normocapnia by increasing airway pressures against increased intra-abdominal pressures can further increase pulmonary vascular resistance. This is worsened when patients are placed in the Trendelenburg position, which is usually requested by surgeons to improve visualization and surgical access. It is important to have a thorough discussion with the surgeons regarding the patient's disease and the surgical plan for optimal management.

FACTOID

Correction of the original intracardiac defect is contraindicated when the increased pulmonary vascular resistance is irreversible. Pregnancy is strongly discouraged in women.

86 JUVENILE IDIOPATHIC ARTHRITIS

Susan Y. Lei, MD

YOUR PATIENT

A 23-year-old female with a history of juvenile idiopathic arthritis (JIA), currently in remission, presents for contracture release in hands.

Physical examination shows a well-appearing 55-kg female with decreased motion in hands bilaterally.

PREOPERATIVE CONSIDERATIONS

Juvenile idiopathic arthritis, also known as juvenile rheumatoid arthritis, is the most common autoimmune disease of childhood and is characterized by chronic joint inflammation. The etiology and pathogenesis are largely unknown. There is a strong genetic predisposition that is very complex, with multiple genes being responsible for disease onset and manifestations. Humoral and cell-mediated immunity are both involved in the pathogenesis of JIA, and T lymphocytes play a central role in releasing proinflammatory cytokines.

The incidence of JIA is about 4-14 cases per 100,000 children annually, with a prevalence of 1-86 per 100,000 children. It is more commonly found in girls than in boys by a ratio of 3:1, but systemic onset occurs with equal frequency in girls and boys. JIA, by definition, is arthritis beginning before age 16, but the age of onset is often much earlier, usually around the age of 1-3 years. Advances in pharmacologic therapy for JIA over the past 20 years have dramatically improved the prognosis and quality of life for these children, and most of them can lead productive lives when the disease is in remission.

JIA is a clinical diagnosis of exclusion, where arthritis must be present in at least one joint for 6 weeks before a diagnosis can be made. The disease onset can be abrupt or insidious and can be characterized by morning stiffness or stiffness after long periods of sitting or inactivity. Children usually do not complain of pain, but parents will notice that the child will stop using the affected joints normally. There are three subsets of JIA. Oligoarticular JIA, accounting for 50% of cases, occurs when fewer than 5 joints are affected, mainly knees. Polyarticular JIA accounts for 20%-40% of JIA cases and affects more than 5 joints, most commonly the small joints of the hands. Systemic-onset JIA, also known as Still's disease, can involve the cervical spine, jaw, hands, hips, and shoulders and is manifested by spiking fevers with a predictable pattern, occurring 1-2 times a day and around the same time every day. The child appears systemically ill. It is also accompanied by an evanescent rash on the trunk and extremities that lasts for a few hours; this rash is typically nonpruritic, macular, and salmon-colored.

There are no recognized diagnostic serologic tests available. On physical examination, there is either intra-articular swelling or limited joint motion with pain, warmth, or erythema of the joint. Preoperative assessment mainly focuses on airway management because JIA involvement of the temporomandibular joint (TMJ) and mandibular joint, which occurs in more than 60% of children, limits mouth opening. As a result, the mandibular growth is stunted, and micrognathia results. MRI and ultrasonography can help detect TMJ disease. Cervical spine involvement can lead to spinal fusion and decreased cervical movement and stiffness. It is important to obtain radiographic images of the cervical spine prior to surgery.

ANESTHETIC MANAGEMENT

- Consider regional anesthesia to avoid airway manipulation. Ankylosis and osteophytes can make epidural and spinal anesthesia difficult to place.
- For general anesthesia, consider awake fiberoptic intubation with mild sedation and adequate local anesthetic to oropharyngeal structures.
- Maintain manual inline cervical stability during intubation and ventilation.
- Consider using a smaller size endotracheal tube in patients with systemic JIA, as cricoarytenoiditis can severely distort the glottis anatomy.
- Use extra padding for all pressure points.
- Maintain anesthesia with sevoflurane.

POSTOPERATIVE CONSIDERATIONS

Pain control is critical in these patients postoperatively. They should resume their medications for JIA as soon as possible so that their disease does not relapse. Early physical therapy is important in helping to maintain their range of motion and muscle strength.

DOs and DON'Ts

✓ Do use awake fiberoptic intubation, if necessary.
✓ Do consider stress dose steroids, if the patient has been taking steroids in the past year.
⊗ Do avoid extending or flexing neck.

SURGICAL CONCERNS

Surgery for contracture release is fairly simple, and recovery is quick. However, some patients may require more extensive surgery, such as total knee replacements and osteotomies. For children undergoing these surgeries, it is important to take into consideration the child's age and whether his or her bones are still growing. For knee replacements, it is important to consider the possibility of needing another joint replacement in 10 to 20 years. The timing often requires a balance between the child's age, the expected life of the replaced joint, and the possible loss of bone and muscle strength if surgery is delayed too long.

FACTOID

There is a high occurrence of autoimmune diseases in the relatives of children with JIA because many of them share the same genes that make them susceptible to autoimmune diseases.

PART 13

PAIN

87 PAIN MANAGEMENT AFTER SCOLIOSIS REPAIR

John M. Saroyan, MD

YOUR PATIENT

A 14-year-old female with idiopathic scoliosis (IS) is seen on postoperative day 0 following a posterior spinal fusion and instrumentation.

PREOPERATIVE CONSIDERATIONS

Idiopathic scoliosis is a chronic spinal condition; between 1% and 3% of older children and adolescents in the United States are diagnosed with it every year, with a greater prevalence among females. This condition is commonly conservatively managed with bracing therapy and physiotherapy; alternatively, as in the patient described here, a surgical approach using pedicle screws and spinal fusion techniques can be used for more severe cases of curve distortion.

POSTOPERATIVE CONSIDERATIONS

Patients require intensive care unit or stepdown monitoring for medical and surgical management immediately following surgery. In addition, most patients require a large amount of opioid to maintain adequate analgesia in the first 24 hours.

- Use an opioid prescription via patient-controlled analgesia (PCA) for the first 48 hours.
- Make a transition to a regularly administered short-acting opioid such as oral morphine or oxycodone *or* a transition to an oral long-acting opioid such as methadone or oxycodone CR in addition to a short-acting opioid as needed for moderate to severe pain on postoperative days 2 and 3.
- Prescribe a taper for the long-acting opioid, if utilized.
- Prescribe oral acetaminophen as needed for mild pain or around the clock for 3 days as an adjuvant during the most severe postoperative pain before changing to as needed for mild pain.
- Schedule inpatient physical therapy in accordance with the orthopedist's recommendation.

DOs and DON'Ts

⊗   Do not prescribe a demand dose via PCA if the patient is not able to utilize it.

✓   Do monitor for sedation and adequate analgesia after the transition to an oral regimen.

⊗   Do not allow the parent to utilize the demand dose of a developmentally normal patient.

✓   Do begin a bowel regimen on postoperative day 1.

CONTROVERSIES

Intravenous ketorolac for analgesia in the postoperative period. In animal models, nonsteroidal anti-inflammatory drugs (NSAIDs) have been shown to inhibit bone metabolism by disrupting prostaglandin synthesis, reducing immune and inflammatory responses, and inhibiting osteoblast cell production. In adults, a significant inhibitory effect on spinal fusion when using ketorolac has been shown. Retrospective studies in adolescents with IS have not shown that postoperative ketorolac within the first 48 hours of surgery significantly influences the development of pseudoarthrosis or other reasons for failed fusion. At the authors' institution, IV ketorolac is started at 48 hours postop (if blood urea nitrogen and creatinine are normal and hemoglobin is stable) to minimize any effect that the NSAID may have on fusion.

OUTPATIENT CONCERNS

Various short- and long-acting opioid analgesics, as well as sedatives, are increasingly prescribed for relief of pain in the adolescent and young adult population, but carry a risk for misuse and diversion. Attention to the amount of medication dispensed and in-person follow-up with the prescriber postoperatively may decrease these concerns for clinicians, patients, and families.

88 POSTOPERATIVE PAIN MANAGEMENT IN SICKLE CELL DISEASE FOR LAPAROSCOPIC CHOLECYSTECTOMY

Mary E. Tresgallo, DNP, MPH, FNP-BC

YOUR PATIENT

A 16-year-old male patient with sickle cell disease is scheduled for a cholecystectomy. He has been having biliary colic for 3 months; recent ultrasonography confirms cholelithiasis. Past medical history is significant for multiple hospitalizations for management of vaso-occlusive crisis (VOC), once for acute chest syndrome (ACS) at age 11, and once for splenectomy at age 3. His home medication regimen includes hydroxyurea, penicillin, and folic acid. His usual site of VOC pain is in his legs, back, and chest. His inpatient pain management regimen during his last VOC hospitalization included a morphine sulfate patient-controlled analgesia (PCA) and nonsteroidal anti-inflammatory medication. He has taken no opioid for the last 6 months.

PREOPERATIVE CONSIDERATIONS

Patients with sickle cell disease (which includes sickle cell anemia [SS], sickle hemoglobin C disease [SC], and the sickle B thalassemias) who undergo surgery are generally considered to be at greater risk for perioperative complications. Vaso-occlusion, which may involve both the micro- and macrovasculature, is the most important pathophysiologic event in sickle cell disease and explains most of its clinical manifestations. Cholelithiasis has been recognized in increasing numbers of pediatric patients with sickle cell disease.

POSTOPERATIVE CONSIDERATIONS

Intensive care unit admission for close respiratory monitoring should be considered if the patient has a history of pulmonary disease (previous episodes of ACS, recurrent pneumonia). Stress of any kind may trigger the onset of a VOC.

- Opioid prescription via PCA should be considered. PCA prescription can include a demand dose (if age appropriate) with or without a continuous infusion and clinician boluses.
- Patients who have chronic pain and who have been on recent standing opioids preoperatively may have developed opioid tolerance and may require higher doses of opioid intra- and postoperatively; they may also be at risk for opioid withdrawal if their standing preoperative opioid dose requirement is not addressed postoperatively.
- Laxatives should be prescribed for patients on opioids to avoid the risk of constipation. Caution should be exercised in the setting of abdominal surgery, and the prescribing of laxatives should be done in concert with surgical team recommendations.
- Acetaminophen at appropriate weight-based doses can be given as an adjuvant for mild breakthrough pain.
- A transition to oral opioids should be considered for postoperative pain control for a patient who has undergone an uncomplicated laparoscopic cholecystectomy once the patient is tolerating oral intake and is able to ambulate.

DOs and DON'Ts

✓   Do consider the co-administration of adjuvants with the primary opioid analgesics to enhance their analgesic potential and obviate or ameliorate opioid side effects if co-administration of adjuvants is not otherwise medically or surgically contraindicated.

⊗   Do not start a continuous infusion via PCA for a laparoscopic cholecystectomy if the patient can execute a demand dose unless there is established opioid tolerance, concurrent VOC, or another compelling reason to do so.

✓   Do monitor for sedation and adequate pain control for the duration of analgesic therapy.

⊗   Do not forget that uncontrolled pain and splinting after thoracic or abdominal surgeries can decrease chest wall motion and lead to regional hypoventilation and atelectasis. This may progress to more severe pulmonary sequelae such as ACS. Conversely, hypoventilation caused by narcotic analgesics may also play a role.

CONTROVERSIES

- Use of preoperative red blood cell transfusion to achieve a hemoglobin S level of less than 30% or a hemoglobin of 10 g/dL in order to decrease the risk of intraoperative and postoperative morbidity and mortality.

- Use of regional anesthesia techniques intraoperatively and/or postoperatively for the management of surgical pain or pain secondary to VOC.

SURGICAL CONCERNS

Perioperative management of hypoxia, hypoperfusion, and acidosis is critical to minimize erythrocyte sickling to prevent vaso-occlusion and organ dysfunction. In doing so, the morbidity and mortality associated with surgery is decreased.

89 INTRAVENOUS PATIENT-CONTROLLED ANALGESIA

Mary E. Tresgallo, DNP, MPH, FNP-BC

YOUR PATIENT

A 15-year-old male is scheduled for an elective colectomy secondary to ulcerative colitis. The family has refused an epidural for postoperative pain management.

PREOPERATIVE CONSIDERATIONS

- Intravenous patient-controlled analgesia (IV PCA) is a method of analgesia administration involving a computer-programmable pump activated by the patient to receive small doses of opioid within defined limits. Titration of the opioid dose should be done after appropriate patient assessment. The settings of the PCA may include a demand dose with a specified lockout interval and a clinician bolus dose at a specified time interval to a maximum dose allowable at a specified frequency, as shown in Table 89.1. A continuous infusion may be prescribed if the patient is unable to push a demand dose button independently or if there is unremitting pain. Cognitively normal children over 8 years old are typically deemed appropriate for a demand dose PCA unless there are other medical or developmental issues.
- IV PCA allows for patients to feel more in control of their pain management.
- Children less than 1 year of age and those with serious medical conditions may have altered pharmacokinetics.
- Be careful with premature infants and infants in general, patients with decreased cardiac output or relative hypoxia (decreased respiratory reserve), patients with a history of central or obstructive sleep apnea, patients who are at risk for increased intracranial pressure, patients with renal or liver insufficiency, patients who are morbidly obese, and patients who have a history of opioid tolerance or dependence or who have a history of hypersensitivity to opioids.

TABLE 89-1   INTRAVENOUS PATIENT CONTROLLED ANALGESIA INITIAL OPIOID INFUSION ORDERS

Drug (and concentrations)	Continuous Basal Infusion,* μg/kg/h (range, μg/kg/h)	Demand Dose, μg/kg (range, μg/kg)	Demand Dose Lockout Interval, Minutes (range)	Number of Demand Doses/Hour (range)	†Clinician Bolus Dose (μg/kg)	†Clinician Bolus Dose Lockout Interval, Minutes (range)
Morphine	10 (10-15)	15 (10-30)	10 (6-20)	6 (1-10)	15 (15-30)	20 (15-30)
Hydromorphone	3 (2-3)	3 (2-6)	10 (6-20)	6 (1-10)	3 (3-6)	20 (15-30)
Fentanyl	0.1 (0.1-0.25)	0.1 (0.05-0.25)	15 (10-20)	4 (1-6)	0.1 (0.05-0.25)	20 (20-30)

*A basal infusion is not always used. It may increase the risk of excessive sedation or respiratory depression.

†The clinician bolus dose (μg/kg) can be administered at the specified lockout interval (minutes) to a maximum dose of 3 doses every 4 hours as needed for break-through pain.

Guidelines are to be followed in an acute care setting; dosages must be individualized for each patient.

POSTOPERATIVE CONSIDERATIONS

- In general, equianalgesic doses of opioid produce similar degrees of respiratory depression, except in premature infants or in patients who have disordered breathing secondary to central or obstructive apnea.
- Sedation typically precedes respiratory depression.
- Patients who are receiving methadone or those with obstructive apnea, or central respiratory control issues may have unpredictable respiratory responses to opioids.
- Patients should always be monitored closely for signs of sedation when opioids are prescribed.
- Patients with chronic pain who have been on opioids preoperatively may be opioid tolerant and require higher doses of opioid intra- and postoperatively; they may also be at risk for opioid withdrawal if preoperative opioid dose requirements are not addressed postoperatively.
- Naloxone is a pure opioid antagonist that is nonselective in its opioid reversal. It reverses the sedation, respiratory, gastrointestinal, and analgesic effects of opioids. Administration must be done with caution, particularly in patients who are opioid dependent, tolerant, or who are in extreme pain, to avoid acute withdrawal symptoms. The usual initial dose of naloxone in children is 0.01 mg/kg; the dose is titrated to achieve the desired effect. Note that naloxone has a plasma half-life elimination of only 60 minutes; this is a much shorter duration of action than the agonist it is used to reverse. Bag mask ventilation may be used to support the patient until respiration reaches an appropriate level.
- Proper assessment and reassessment of pain after an intervention is the cornerstone of optimal pain management. A developmentally appropriate pain scale should be utilized.
- Postoperative pain management requires the appropriate infrastructure, including relevant policies, procedures, and protocols to ensure the appropriate and safe monitoring of patients.

DOs and DON'Ts

✓   Do consider the administration of co-analgesic adjuvants such as nonsteroidal anti-inflammatory drugs (NSAIDs) to enhance pain control and for their opioid-sparing effects. Postoperative muscular spasms can be treated with diazepam 0.01- 0.05 mg/kg every 8 hours (PO preferred over IV administration).

✓   Do prescribe medication for potential side effects related to postoperative PCA opioid administration (antiemetics and antipruritics). A low-dose intravenous infusion of naloxone

(0.25-1 µg/kg/h) or the partial agonist/antagonist nalbuphine (50 µg/kg, maximum 5 mg/dose) is an effective alternative for treating opioid-induced pruritus rather than prescribing antihistamines.

✓   Do prescribe a bowel regimen to minimize the risk of constipation; this is easier to prevent than to treat. Caution should be exercised in the setting of abdominal surgery and the prescribing of a bowel regimen should be done after consultation with the surgical team.

✓   Do prescribe a continuous infusion if you expect unremitting pain despite adequate use of demand boluses or for patients who are unable to press the button.

✓   Close clinical monitoring is necessary in pediatric patients with a PCA. In general, continuous pulse oximetry is employed. This cannot replace frequent clinical nursing assessment of the patient.

✓   Do exercise caution with the administration of other respiratory or central nervous system depressant medications, especially the commonly used antihistamines and benzodiazepines, due to increased risk of sedation when the patient is receiving a concomitant opioid.

⊗   Do not prescribe IV PCA in a patient who has mental status changes or is otherwise medically unstable.

CONTROVERSIES

• PCA by proxy (with a parent or surrogate as proxy) is extremely controversial, since it bypasses the inherent safety of the patient's not pushing for the next demand dose if there is sedation present. A safer option may be nurse-controlled analgesia, where the nurse can give clinician boluses via the PCA after appropriate patient assessment.

SURGICAL CONSIDERATIONS

Patients on PCA require diligent and regular assessment of their medical and surgical condition. A complaint of pain mandates appropriate patient assessment, not a reflexive increase in the amount of opioid prescribed.

FACTOID

Patients who are able to play a video game using complex visual motor skills are usually able to grasp the concept of a PCA pump.

APPENDIX 1
PEDIATRIC ANESTHESIOLOGY SUGGESTED DRUG DOSAGES

Drugs and dosage are intended as general guidelines ONLY. Adjust dosages based on clinical situation: hepatorenal function, cardiopulmonary bypass, extracorporeal membrane oxygenation (ECMO), and other factors.

RESUSCITATION MEDICATION

Atropine: 0.01-0.03 mg/kg IM, IV, ET, IC, IO

Sodium bicarbonate: 1-2 mEq/kg ($0.3 \times$ kg $\times$ BE) IV, IC, IO

Calcium chloride 10-30 mg/kg IV, IC slowly (max 1 g/dose)

Calcium gluconate 60-100 mg/kg IV, IC (max 2 g/dose)

Dextrose 0.5-1 g/kg IV = 1-2 mL/kg D_{50}; or 2-4 mL/kg $D_{25}W$ or 5-10 mL/kg $D_{10}W$ or 10-20 mL/kg D_5NS

Diltiazem (Cardizem): 0.25 mg/kg over 2 min; may repeat in 15 min @ 0.35 mg/kg over 2 min

Ephedrine: 0.2-0.3 mg/kg/dose

Epinephrine 10 μg/kg IV, IC, IO; ET = 100 μg/kg

Lidocaine: 1 mg/kg IV, IC, ET, IO

Lipid emulsion (Intralipid): 20% 1.5 mL/kg over 1 min × 3 prn, 0.25 mL/kg/min then 0.5 mL/kg/min if hypotensive

DEFIBRILLATION/CARDIOVERSION

V-Fib: 2 J/kg then 4 J/kg (defibrillation = unsynchronized) using the largest paddles that fit

Synchronized cardioversion: 0.5-1 then 2 J/kg

Adenosine: 0.1 mg/kg IV push (max 6 mg); repeat 0.2 mg/kg (max 12 mg)

CARDIAC

Amiodarone: V Fib: 5 mg/kg IV load over 30 sec (max 300 mg)
SVT: 5 mg/kg over 10 min × 5 doses; non-PVC container

Digoxin: initial load 4-25 μg/kg IV Maintenance 5-10 μg/kg/dose BID
IV dose = 2/3 PO dose

Diltiazem: 0.25 mg/kg over 2 min; may repeat in 15 min @ 0.35 mg/kg over 2 min

Dopamine, dobutamine: 2-20 μg/kg/min

Ephedrine: 0.2-0.3 mg/kg/dose

Epinephrine, isoproterenol, norepinephrine: 0.05-1 μg/kg/min

Esmolol: 0.5 mg/kg bolus over 1 min; Maintenance: 50-300 μg/kg/min

Lidocaine: 1-2 mg/kg/dose IV 20-50 μg/kg/min (adult dose 1-4 mg/min)

Magnesium sulfate for torsades de pointes: 25-50 mg/kg (max 2 g) over 10-20 min

Milrinone: 20-50 μg/kg load; maintenance: 0.3-0.7 μg/kg/min

Nitroglycerin: 0.5-5 μg/kg/min

Nitroprusside: 0.5-10 μg/kg/min

PGE_1 = Alprostadil: 0.05-0.1 μg/kg/min

Phenylephrine: 0.5-10 μg/kg/min; 1 μg/kg bolus

Procainamide: 3-6 mg/kg (max 100 mg each dose) over 5 min × 3 q 5-10 min
Maintenance: 20-80 μg/kg/min (adult 1-4 mg/min)

Propranolol: 0.05-0.15 mg/kg IV slowly (max 5 mg)

Vasopressin: Mix 10 U in 50 mL so 1 mL = 0.2 U
hypotension: 0.0005-0.002 U/kg/min
GI bleed: 0.002-0.005 U/kg/min

Verapamil: 0.05-0.2 mg/kg IV over 2 min (max 5 mg)

MUSCLE RELAXANTS

Cisatracurium: 0.1-0.2 mg/kg/dose IV; lasts 15-45 min

Pancuronium: 0.1 mg/kg/dose IV; lasts 1-2 h

Rocuronium: 0.4-1.0 mg/kg/dose IV; 0.6 mg/kg/h

Succinylcholine: 1-2 mg/kg IV; 4 mg/kg IM; consider giving atropine first

Vecuronium: 0.1 mg/kg/dose IV; 60 μg/kg/h

SEDATIVE/IV ANESTHETICS

Chloral hydrate: 30-80 mg/kg/dose PO, PR

Clonidine: 0.004 mg/kg PO (max 0.1 mg)

Dexmedetomidine: load with 1 μg/kg IV over 5 min, then 0.2-1 μg/kg/h

Diphenhydramine: 0.2-2 mg/kg/dose IV q4-6h; or 1.25 mg/kg/dose q6h (max 400 mg/d)

Etomidate: 0.3 mg/kg IV

Haloperidol: 1-3 mg IM for pt. >6 years

Ketamine: 1-2 mg/kg IV; 3-6 mg/kg PO; 6-10 mg/kg PR; 3 mg/kg intranasal

Methohexital: 1-2 mg/kg/dose IV; 30-40 mg/kg PR

Midazolam: 0.05-0.3 mg/kg IV, IM;
Infusion: 0.4 μg/kg/min
PO: 0.5-0.75 mg/kg

Midazolam (*continued*)

PR: 0.5-1 mg/kg

Intranasal: 0.2 mg/kg

Pentobarbital: 2 mg/kg IM, IV, PO

Propofol: 2-3 mg/kg IV
Maintenance: 50-300 µg/kg/min

Thiopental: 3-7 mg/kg IV; PR: 20-40 mg/kg

ANALGESICS

NSAIDs

Acetaminophen: PO 10-15 mg/kg q4h

PR (1st dose only) 30-40 mg/kg, next PO dose 6 h later
max 30 mg/kg/d in newborns
max 60 mg/kg/d in infants
max 90 mg/kg/d in children
max 4 g/d in adults

Ibuprofen: 10 mg/kg PO q6h

Ketorolac: 0.5 mg/kg IV q6h (max 30 mg) normal creat and no bleeding
diathesis; max 120 mg/d; max 5 days

OPIOIDS

Codeine: 0.5-1.0 mg/kg PO q4h

Tylenol #1: acetaminophen 300 mg + codeine 7.5 mg

Tylenol #2: acetaminophen 300 mg + codeine 15 mg

Tylenol #3: acetaminophen 300 mg + codeine 30 mg

Tylenol #4: acetaminophen 300 mg + codeine 60 mg

Fentanyl: 0.5-1 µg/kg/dose IV q1h prn

Hydrocodone/oxycodone: 0.05-0.15 mg/kg PO q4h (usual start dose 0.1 mg/kg)

Hydromorphone: 0.03 mg/kg PO q4h; 0.015 mg/kg IV q2-4h prn

Meperidine: for rigors 0.1 mg/kg IV once

Methadone: sliding scale:
Mild pain: 25 µg/kg IV q4h prn
Moderate pain: 50 µg/kg IV q4h prn
Severe pain: 75 µg/kg IV q4h prn or as a long-acting opioid 0.1 mg/kg q8-12h
  (beware of cumulative effects after 48-72 h)

Morphine: 0.05-0.15 mg/kg IV q2-4h prn; 0.3-0.5 mg/kg/dose PO q4h

Remifentanil: 0.1-0.5 µg/kg/min, 1-4 µg/kg bolus

Sufentanil: 10-25 µg/kg induction

REVERSALS

Neostigmine 0.05 mg/kg with glycopyrrolate 0.01 mg/kg (or with atropine 0.02 mg/kg)

Edrophonium: for myasthenia: 0.2 mg/kg IV
NMB reversal: 1 mg/kg IV with atropine 0.014 mg/kg

Flumazenil: sedation reversal: 0.01 mg/kg IV q 1 min
Overdose: 0.01 mg/kg q 1 min or 0.005-0.01 mg/kg/h (max 0.2 mg/dose; cumulative max 1 mg)

Naloxone: 0.01-0.1 mg/kg/dose IV, ET; lasts 20 min

Physostigmine: 0.01 mg/kg slowly IV (adult dose 2 mg) with atropine 0.01-0.02 mg/kg

FLUIDS/ELECTROLYTES/DIURETICS

Maintenance: 4 mL/kg/h for 1st 10 kg + 2 mL/kg/h for 2nd 10 kg + 1 mL/kg/h for every kg >20 kg

Calcium: 200-300 mEq/kg/d

Furosemide: 0.5-1 mg/kg PO, IV; 0.06-0.24 mg/kg/h

Glucose: 8 mg/kg/min

Hyperkalemia: Dextrose 1 g/kg IV over 15 min with 0.2 U reg insulin/g dextrose;
Ca^{++} = 4-5 mg/kg IV over 5-10 min;
Kayexalate: 1-2 g/kg PO, PR (with 20% sorbitol)

Magnesium sulfate: 25-50 mg/kg (max 2 g) over 10 min; maintenance: 16 mg/kg/h to achieve plasma levels of 0.8-1.2 mmol/L (max 2 g)

Mannitol: 0.25-1 g/kg IV

Potassium: 2-3 mEq/kg/d

PRBC: 10 mL/kg will raise Hg by 1 g

Platelets: 5-10 mL/kg will raise count 50-100 × 10^9/L; for >10 kg patient, 1 U/10 kg

Shock: 10-20 mL/kg of NS, RL, or 5% albumin

Sodium bicarbonate = $NaHCO_3$ = 1-2 mEq/kg

Vasopressin for diabetes insipidus: 0.0005 U/kg/h double q 30 min up to 0.01 U/kg/h, dilute to 0.04 U/mL

ANTIBIOTICS

Ampicillin: 25-50 mg/kg q4-6h (max 2 g)

Cefazolin: 30 mg/kg IV q4h (max 2 g)

Cefoxitin: 30 mg/kg IV q4h (max 2 g)

Clindamycin: 10 mg/kg q6h (max 900 mg) over 30 min

Gentamicin: 2 mg/kg (max 80 mg) over 30 min, no redose

Metronidazole: 7.5 mg/kg IV q6h over 30 min; (max 500 mg)

Tobramycin 2.5 mg/kg (max 200 mg) over 30 min q8h

Unasyn: 75 mg/kg IV over 30 min q4h

Vancomycin: 15 mg/kg over 60 min q6-8h

Zosyn: <9 mos: 240 mg/kg/d divide q6-8h

>9 mos: 300 mg/kg/d divide q6-8h

ANTIHYPERTENSIVES

Esmolol: 0.5 mg/kg bolus over 1 min; maintenance: 50-300 µg/kg/min

Hydralazine: 0.1-0.2 mg/kg IM, IV q4-6h

Labetalol: 0.25 mg/kg IV q1-2h

Nifedipine: 0.01-0.02 mg/kg IV or 1-2 mg/kg/d
PO, SL (adult dose 10-30 mg PO)

Phentolamine: 0.1 mg/kg/dose IV

Propranolol: 0.01-0.15 mg/kg IV slowly

ANTIEMETICS/H2 BLOCKERS

Granisetron: 10 µg/kg/dose IV/PO q12h

Metoclopramide (Reglan): 0.1 mg/kg IV/PO q6h (caution re: extrapyramidal signs)

Esomeprazole (Nexium): 1 mg/kg IV QD (max 40 mg)

Ondansetron: 0.15 mg/kg IV/SL/PO q8h slowly (max 8 mg/dose; 32 mg/d)

Prochlorperazine (Compazine): >2 y 0.1 mg/kg/dose
IV/PO q8h (caution re: extrapyramidal signs)

Ranitidine (Zantac): 1-2 mg/kg/dose BID PO, IV (max 150 mg BID)

STEROIDS

Dexamethasone: 0.3-1 mg/kg IV (for ENT 0.5 mg/kg, max 10 mg)

Hydrocortisone (Solu-Cortef): 0.2-1 mg/kg q6h (anti-inflammatory); status
asthmaticus: load 4-8 mg/kg then 2-4 mg/kg q4-6h

Methylprednisolone (Solu-Medrol): 0.04-0.2 mg/kg q6h (anti-inflammatory);
status asthmaticus: load 2 mg/kg, then 0.5-1 mg/kg/dose q4-6h
spinal shock: 30 mg/kg IV over 1 h, then 5.4 mg/kg/h × 23 h
liver transplantation: 20 mg/kg

ANTIPRURITICS

Diphenhydramine: 0.5 mg/kg/dose PO/IV q6h

Hydroxyzine: 0.5 mg/kg/dose PO/IV q6h

Nalbuphine: 0.1 mg/kg/dose q6h IV over 20 min (max 5 mg)

BRONCHODILATORS

Albuterol nebulizer (0.5% soln): 0.01 mL/kg/2.5 mL NS (max 0.5 mL = 2.5 mg)

Aminophylline: 7 mg/kg slowly over 30 min IV; maintenance: 0.5-1.5 mg/kg/h

Epinephrine (1:1,000): 10 μg/kg SC (max 400 μg)
Racemic epi: 0.25-0.5 mL/5 mL NS nebulized

Isoproterenol: 0.05 μg/kg/min increasing by 0.1 μg/kg/min to effect or too tachycardic

Metaproterenol nebulizer (5% soln): 0.01 mL/kg/2.5 mL NS (max dose 0.3 mL = 15 mg)

Terbutaline 10 μg/kg SC (max 250 μg)

PCA

Hydromorphone (0.2 mg/mL):
  Demand: 0.003 mg/kg/dose q10min
  Cont. infusion (optional): 0.003 mg/kg/h
  Clinician boluses: 0.006 mg/kg q20min up to 3 times q4h

Morphine (1 mg/mL); if under 10 kg (0.5 mg/mL):
  Demand: 0.015 mg/kg q10min
  Cont. infusion (optional): 0.015 mg/kg/h
  Clinician boluses: 0.03 mg/kg q20min up to 3 times q4h

EPIDURAL

Bupivacaine 0.1% (1 mg/mL ± fentanyl 1-2 μg/mL ± clonidine 0.1 μg/mL): 0.1-0.4 ml/kg/h

Do not exceed:
Neonates: 0.2 mg/kg/h of bupivacaine, no longer than 48 h

Older children: 0.4 mg/kg/h of bupivacaine

Caudal (single shot): 0.25% bupivacaine (± epi premixed) 0.75-1 mL/kg ± clonidine 1 μg/kg

MISCELLANEOUS

Aminocaproic acid:

Cardiac: 200 mg/kg, then 16.7 mg/kg/h, max 18 g/m^2/d
Ortho: 100-150 mg/kg, then 10-15 mg/kg/h, max 18/m^2/d

Dantrolene: 2.5 mg/kg IV load; repeat until signs of MH are reversed; up to 30 mg/kg may be necessary
Maintenance: 1.2 mg/kg IV q6h as needed

Heparin: 50-100 U/kg IV bolus, then 10-20 U/kg/h; cardiopulmonary bypass: 300 U/kg IV

Insulin: 0.02-0.1 U/kg/h

Factor VIIa: 40 μg/kg IV, redose 90 min later with 90 μg/kg IV, then redose 2 h later with 90 μg/kg

ET = endotracheal; IC = intracardiac; IM = intramuscular; IO = intraosseous; IV = intravenous; PO = oral; PR = rectal; SC = subcutaneous; μg = microgram

APPENDIX 2
PEDIATRIC SIZING CHART

PEDIATRIC SIZING CHART

Age- and Weight-Based Sizing Chart

Age (or Weight)	Uncuffed ETT	Cuffed ETT	Laryngoscope Blade	DL ETT	CVL	A-line	LMA	Foley	Chest Tube	Salem Sump
1 kg	2.5		Miller 00		5 Fr	24 G	1	5 Fr	8 Fr	
2 kg	3		Miller 00		5 Fr	24 G	1	5 Fr	10 Fr	10 Fr
3 kg	3		Miller 0		5 Fr	24 G	1	5 Fr	12 Fr	10 Fr
Term newborn	3.5		Miller 1		5 Fr	24 G	1	5 Fr	12 Fr	10 Fr
5 kg	3.5		Miller 1		5 Fr	24 G	1.5	5 Fr	12 Fr	10 Fr
1 year	4		Miller 1		5 Fr	24 G	1.5	5 Fr	16 Fr	10 Fr
2 years	4.5		Miller/Mac 2		5 Fr	24 G	2	8 Fr	16 Fr	14 Fr
3 years	4.5		Miller/Mac 2		5 Fr	22 G	2	8 Fr	20 Fr	14 Fr
4 years	5		Miller/Mac 2		5 Fr	22 G	2	8 Fr	20 Fr	14 Fr
5 years		5	Miller/Mac 2		5 Fr	22 G	2	8 Fr	20 Fr	14 Fr
6 years		5	Miller/Mac 2		7 Fr	22 G	2.5	8 Fr	20 Fr	14 Fr
7 years		5	Miller/Mac 2		7 Fr	22 G	2.5	8 Fr	20 Fr	14 Fr
8 years		5.5	Miller/Mac 2	26 Fr	7 Fr	22 G	2.5	8 Fr	20 Fr	14 Fr
9 years		5.5	Miller/Mac 2	26 Fr	7 Fr	22 G	2.5	10 Fr	20 Fr	14 Fr

(Continued)

PEDIATRIC SIZING CHART (*Continued*)

Age- and Weight-Based Sizing Chart

Age (or Weight)	Uncuffed ETT	Cuffed ETT	Laryngoscope Blade	DL ETT	CVL	A-line	LMA	Foley	Chest Tube	Salem Sump
10 years		6	Miller/Mac 3	28 Fr	7 Fr	20 G	2.5	10 Fr	20 Fr	14 Fr
11 years		6	Miller/Mac 3	28 Fr	7 Fr	20 G	3	10 Fr	24 Fr	14 Fr
12 years		6	Miller/Mac 3	28 Fr	7 Fr	20 G	3	10 Fr	24 Fr	14 Fr
13 years		6	Miller/Mac 3	32 Fr	9 Fr	20 G	3	12 Fr	24 Fr	16 Fr
14 years		7	Miller/Mac 3	32 Fr	9 Fr	20 G	3	12 Fr	32 Fr	16 Fr
15 years		7	Miller/Mac 3	35 Fr	9 Fr	20 G	4	12 Fr	32 Fr	16 Fr
16 years		7	Miller/Mac 3	35 Fr	9 Fr	20 G	4	12 Fr	32 Fr	16 Fr
17 years		7	Miller/Mac 3	35 Fr	9 Fr	20 G	4	12 Fr	36 Fr	16 Fr
18 years		7	Miller/Mac 3	35 Fr	9 Fr	20 G	4	12 Fr	36 Fr	16 Fr

DL, double-lumen; ETT, endotracheal tube; Fr, French; G, gauge LMA, laryngeal mask airway.

ETT depth (cm) = three times ETT size (mm ID).

ETT size (mm ID) = (age [in years])/4 + 4.

APPENDIX 3

PEDIATRIC CRITICAL EVENTS CHECKLISTS

Reprinted with permission from the Society for Pediatric Anesthesia. Please refer to the following site for any updates to the checklist: http://www.pedsanesthesia.org/newnews/Critical_Event_Checklists.pdf

AIR EMBOLISM
($\downarrow$ETCO$_2$ $\downarrow$SaO$_2$ $\downarrow$BP)

Objective: Restore normal SpO$_2$, hemodynamic stability, and stop source of air entry.

✓ **Call for help. Notify surgeon.**
✓ Increase **oxygen to 100%.**
✓ **Stop** nitrous oxide and volatile agents.
✓ Find **air entry point, stop source, and limit further entry.**
  - Flood wound with irrigation.
  - Check for open venous lines or air in tubing.
  - Turn off all pressurized gas sources (laparoscope, endoscope).
  - Lower surgical site below level of heart (if possible).
  - Perform Valsalva on patient using hand ventilation.
  - Compress jugular veins intermittently if head or cranial case.
  - Left side down once source controlled.
✓ Consider:
  - Vasopressors (epinephrine, norepinephrine).
  - **Chest compressions:** 100/min; to force air through lock, even if not in cardiac arrest.
✓ Call for **transesophageal echocardiography** (if available and/or diagnosis unclear).

ANAPHYLAXIS
(RASH, BRONCHOSPASM, HYPOTENSION)

✓ **Call for help.**
✓ **Increase oxygen to 100%.**
✓ Remove suspected trigger(s).
  • If latex is suspected, thoroughly wash area.
✓ Ensure adequate ventilation/oxygenation.
✓ Obtain IV access.
✓ If hypotensive, turn off anesthetic agents.
✓ Rapidly infuse NS or LR (10-30 mL/kg IV) to restore intravascular volume.
✓ **Epinephrine** (1-10 µg/kg IV as needed) to restore BP and ↓ mediator release.
  • Epinephrine infusion (0.02-0.2 µg/kg/min) may be required to maintain BP.
✓ Adjuvants
  • Beta-agonists (**albuterol** 4-10 puffs as needed) for broncho-constriction.
  • **Methylprednisolone** (2 mg/kg IV, max 100 mg) to ↓ mediator release.
  • **Diphenhydramine** (1 mg/kg IV, max 50 mg) to ↓ histamine-mediated effects.
  • **Famotidine** (0.25 mg/kg IV) or **ranitidine** (1 mg/kg IV) to ↓ effects of histamine.
✓ If anaphylactic reaction requires laboratory confirmation, send mast cell tryptase level within 2 hours of event.

COMMON CAUSATIVE AGENTS

Neuromuscular blockers, latex, chlorhexidine, IV colloids, antibiotics

BRADYCARDIA: UNSTABLE
(BRADYCARDIA ± HEART BLOCK, HYPOTENSIVE WITH PULSES)

Age < 30 days: HR < 100
Age > 30 days < 1 year: HR < 80
Age > 1 year: HR < 60

✓ **Call for help and transcutaneous pacer.**
✓ **Hypoxia is common cause of bradycardia.**
  - Ensure pt is not hypoxic. Give 100% oxygen.
  - Go to "Hypoxia" card if hypoxia persists.
✓ **Stop surgical** stimulation. If laparoscopy, desufflate.
✓ Consider:
  - **Epinephrine** 2-10 µg/kg IV.
  - **Chest compression** if ↓ pulses.
  - **Atropine** (0.01-0.02 mg/kg IV) if vagal etiology.
✓ Assess for drug-induced causes.
  - Beta-blocker overdose: **Glucagon** 0.05 mg/kg IV, then 0.07 mg/kg/h IV infusion.
  - Calcium channel blocker overdose: **Calcium chloride** 10-20 mg/kg IV or **calcium gluconate 50 mg/kg,** then glucagon if calcium ineffective.
✓ **If PEA develops, start chest compressions. Go to "Cardiac Arrest: Asystole, PEA"**

INSTRUCTIONS FOR PACING

1. Place pacing ECG electrodes **AND** pacer pads on chest per package instructions.
2. Turn monitor/defibrillator ON, set to PACER mode.
3. Set PACER RATE (ppm) to desired rate/min. (Can be adjusted up or down based on clinical response once pacing is established.)
4. Increase the milliamperes (mA) of PACER OUTPUT until electrical capture (pacer spikes aligned with QRS complex; threshold normally 65-100 mA).
5. Set final mA to 10 mA above this level.
6. Confirm pulse present.

CARDIAC ARREST: ASYSTOLE, PEA
(NONSHOCKABLE AND/OR PULSELESS CARDIAC ARREST)

✓ **Call for help.**
✓ Designate team leader, assign roles.
✓ Give 100% oxygen. Turn off all anesthetic gases and infusions. Place pt on backboard.
✓ Obtain defibrillator.
✓ **Start chest compressions (100 chest compressions/min + 8 breaths/min).**
  • Maintain good hand position.
  • Maximize $ETCO_2$ > 10 mm Hg with force/depth of compressions.
  • Allow full recoil between compressions.
  • Switch with another provider every 2 minutes, if possible.
  • Use sudden increase in $ETCO_2$ for ROSC—do not stop compressions for pulse check.
✓ **Epinephrine** 10 µg/kg IV q3-5min.
✓ Check pulse & rhythm (q2min during compressor switch).
✓ No pulse and not shockable: resume CPR and checklist.

Read Out H & Ts

Hypovolemia	Tension pneumothorax
Hypoxemia	Tamponade (cardiac)
Hydrogen ion (acidosis)	Thrombosis
Hyperkalemia	Toxin (anesthetic, β-blocker)
Hypoglycemia	Trauma (bleeding outside surgical area)
Hypothermia	

✓ Call for ECMO (if available) if no ROSC after 6 min of CPR.
✓ **Notify parents/guardian that cardiac arrest occurred.**

CARDIAC ARREST: VF/VT
(SHOCKABLE, PULSELESS CARDIAC ARREST)

✓ **Call for help and defibrillator.**
✓ Designate team leader/assign roles.

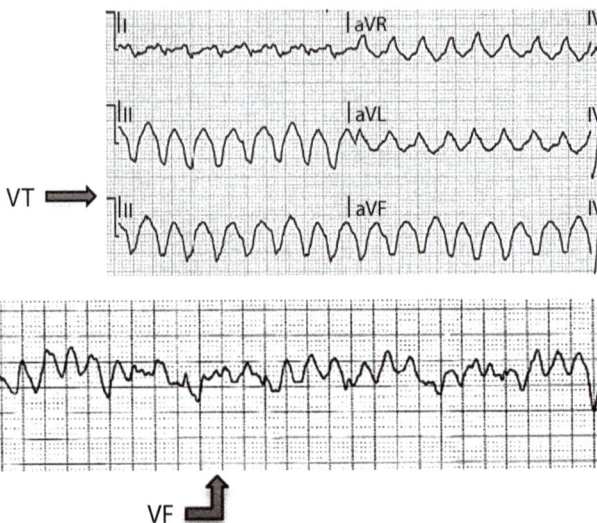

✓ Give 100% oxygen. Turn off all anesthetic gases. Place pt on backboard.
✓ **Start chest compressions (100 chest compressions/min + 8 breaths/min).**
  • Maintain good hand position.
  • Maximize $ETCO_2$ >10 mm Hg with force/depth of compressions.
  • Allow full recoil between compressions—lift hands off chest.
✓ **Shock** 2-4 J/kg.
✓ Resume chest compressions × 2 min.
✓ **Epinephrine** 10 μg/kg IV.
✓ Check pulse and rhythm (q2min during compressor switch).

IF SHOCKABLE RHYTHM CONTINUES

✓ **Shock** 4 J/kg.
✓ Resume chest compressions × 2 min.
✓ **Epinephrine** 10 μg/kg IV.
✓ Check pulse and rhythm (q2min during compressor switch).
✓ **Shock** 4-10 J/kg, continue chest compressions, and epinephrine 10 μg/kg every 3-5 min.
✓ **Amiodarone** 5 mg/kg bolus; may repeat × 2.
✓ Call for **ECMO** (if available) after 6 min of CPR.
✓ Notify parents/guardian that cardiac arrest occurred.

CARDIAC ARREST: PRONE CPR
(CHEST COMPRESSION FOR PATIENT IN PRONE POSITION)

✓ **Call for help.**

CHILDREN/ADOLESCENTS

No Midline Incision:

Compress with heel of hand on spine and second hand on top.

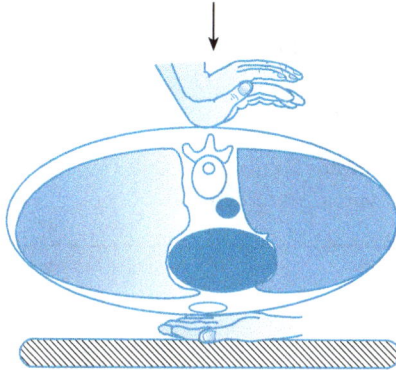

From: Dequin P-F et al. Cardiopulmonary resuscitation in the prone position: Kouwenhoven revisited. *Intensive Care Med.* 1996;22(11):1272.

Midline Incision:

Compress with heel of each hand under scapula.

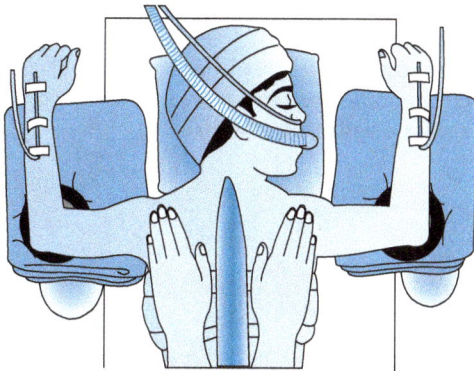

From: Tobias JD et al. Intraoperative cardiopulmonary resuscitation in the prone position. *J Pediatr Surg.* 1994;29(12):1537-1538.

INFANTS

Compress with encircling technique:
- Thumbs midline if no incision.
- Thumbs lateral if incision.

DIFFICULT AIRWAY: AFTER INDUCTION
(UNABLE TO INTUBATE OR VENTILATE; OXYGEN SATURATION < 90%)

✓ **Call for help.**
✓ **Increase oxygen to 100%.**
✓ **Get airway cart.**
✓ **Bag-mask** ventilation.
✓ Notify surgeon—may need to stop or cancel surgery. May awaken if surgery not started.
✓ If unable to mask ventilate, 2-hand if needed:
- Add **oral airway.**
- Add nasal airway.
- Add **LMA.**
✓ Regain spontaneous ventilation, if able.
✓ Alternative approaches for intubation:

• Different blade	• Video-laryngoscope
• Different operator	• Intubating LMA
• Reposition head	• Fiberoptic scope
• Blind oral	• Light wand
• Blind nasal	• Elastic bougie
	• Intubating stylet
	• Retrograde intubation

✓ **If still unable to ventilate:**
- Consider possibility of invasive airway in early stage.
- Emergency noninvasive airway (rigid bronchoscopy).
- **Emergency invasive/surgical airway.**

AIRWAY FIRE
(FIRE IN TRACHEAL TUBE, CIRCUIT, CANISTER)

✓ **Call for help.**
✓ **Disconnect** breathing circuit and **REMOVE** ETT.
✓ **Stop** all gas flow (O_2, N_2O).
✓ Pour saline into airway.
✓ Remove sponges and other flammable materials from airway.
✓ Reintubate and reestablish ventilation.
✓ If intubation difficult, don't hesitate to obtain surgical airway.
✓ Consider bronchoscopy to assess for thermal injury, look for tracheal tube fragments, and remove residual material.
✓ Impound all equipment and supplies for later inspection.

OR FIRE: NONAIRWAY

(FIRE IN OR, EQUIPMENT, SMOKE, ODOR, FLASH/FIRE ON PATIENT)

✓ **Call for help.**
✓ **Protect patient, contain fire.**
✓ If drapes on fire, **remove drapes** from patient.
✓ **Activate fire alarm.**
✓ **Stop medical gases.**
✓ Declare team leader and define roles.
✓ Make one attempt to extinguish fire.
  • Use fire extinguisher or saline-soaked gauze.
✓ If fire not extinguished on first attempt:
  • Remove patient from OR.
  • Confine fire by closing all OR doors.
  • Turn off O_2 gas supply to OR.
✓ Impound all equipment and supplies for later inspection.

HYPERKALEMIA
(SERUM K⁺ > 6 mEq/L)

CAUSES

✓ Excessive intake: massive or "old" blood transfusion, cardioplegia, "K⁺ runs."
✓ Shift of K⁺ from tissues to plasma: crush injury, burns, succinylcholine, malignant hyperthermia, acidosis.
✓ Inadequate excretion: renal failure.

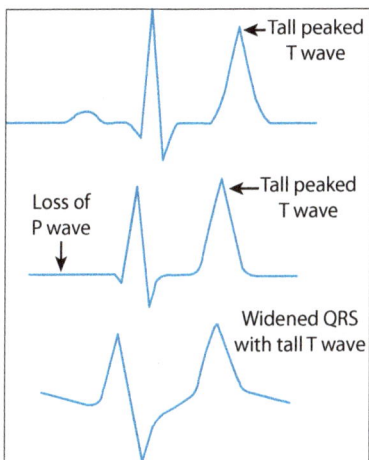

From: Slovis C, Jenkins R. ABC of clinical electrocardiography: conditions not primarily affecting the heart. *BMJ*. 2002;324(7349):1320-1323.

MANIFESTATIONS

Tall-peaked T wave, heart block, sine wave, v fib, or asystole

MANAGEMENT

✓ **CALL FOR HELP!**
✓ **Stop K⁺-containing fluids (LR/RBCs) ⇒ Switch to NS/washed RBCs.**
✓ If **hemodynamically unstable:** initiate **CPR/PALS.**
✓ **Hyperventilate with 100% oxygen and give:**
  • **Calcium chloride 20 mg/kg or calcium gluconate 60 mg/kg IV.**
  • Albuterol by inhaler or nebulizer.
  • Insulin IV/SC 0.1 U/kg with dextrose IV 0.25-1 g/kg.
  • Sodium bicarbonate IV 1-2 mEq/kg.
  • Furosemide IV 0.1 mg/kg.
  • Terbutaline 10 µg/kg load, then 0.1-10 µg/kg/min.
✓ **Dialysis** if refractory to treatment.
✓ Activate ECMO (if available) if cardiac arrest > 6 min.

ACUTE HYPERTENSION
(BP > 99TH %TILE FOR AGE + 5 mm Hg)

✓   Consider likely cause. Rule out medication error, light anesthesia, measurement error (eg, transducer level), and other patient-specific factors.

✓   Ensure that correct BP cuff size is used with a cuff bladder width approximately 40% of limb circumference.

✓   99th %tile for BP is based on patient age and height.

Action	Drug (IV Dosing)
Direct smooth muscle relaxation	• **Sodium nitroprusside** 0.5-10 µg/kg/min • **Hydralazine** 0.1-0.2 mg/kg (adult dose 5-10 mg)
β-Adrenergic blockade	• **Esmolol** 100-500 µg/kg over 5 min, then 50-200 µg/kg/min • **Labetalol** (also α effect) 0.2-1 mg/kg q10min or 0.4-3 mg/kg/h (adult dose) • **Propranolol** 10-100 µg/kg slow push (adult dose 1-5 mg)
α_2-Agonist	• **Clonidine** 0.5-2 µg/kg
Calcium channel blockade	• **Nicardipine** 0.5-5 µg/kg/min • **Clevidipine** 0.5-3.5 µg/kg/min
D-1 agonist	• **Fenoldopam** 0.3-0.5 µg/kg/min (max 2.5 µg/kg/min)

Age (y)	99th %tile Systolic Range (5th-95th %tile height)	99th %tile Diastolic Range (5th-95th %tile height)
1	105-114	61-66
2	109-117	66-71
3	111-120	71-75
4	113-122	74-79
5	115-123	77-82
6	116-125	80-84
7	117-126	82-86
8	119-127	83-88
9	120-129	84-89
10	122-130	85-90
11	124-132	86-90
12	126-135	86-91

HYPOTENSION

(<5TH % TILE FOR AGE FOR PT > 1 YEAR, 5TH % TILE = 70 mm Hg + [2 × AGE IN YEARS])

CAUSES OF HYPOTENSION

↓ Preload	↓ Contractility	↓ Afterload
• Hypovolemia • Vasodilation • Impaired venous return • Tamponade • Pulmonary embolism	• Negative inotropic drugs (anesthetic agents) • Arrhythmias • Hypoxemia • Heart failure (ischemia)	• Drug-induced vasodilation • Sepsis • Anaphylaxis • Endocrine crisis

TREATMENT OF HYPOTENSION

✓ Inform surgeon and OR nurse.
✓ Ensure oxygenation/ventilation.
✓ Turn off anesthetic agents.
✓ Verify patient is truly hypotensive; check cuff size and position.

✓ Expand circulating blood volume (administer fluids rapidly). ✓ Trendelenburg position. ✓ Place or replace IV; consider interosseous needle.	✓ Start inotrope infusion (dopamine, epinephrine, milrinone) as needed. ✓ Review ECG for rhythm disturbances or ischemia. ✓ Send ABG, Hb, electrolytes.	✓ Start vasopressor infusion: phenylephrine, norepinephrine. ✓ Follow "Anaphylaxis" card if appropriate. ✓ Administer steroids for endocrine crisis.

HYPOXIA
($\downarrow$SpO$_2$ $\downarrow$PaO$_2$)

Hypoxia: All Patients	Hypoxia: Intubated Patients
Give 100% oxygen Check: ✓ Oxygen flow ✓ Airway patency ✓ Breathing circuit connected and patent ✓ Ventilation rate and depth adequate ✓ Listen to breath sounds: • Wheezing • Crackles • Diminished or absent ✓ Is pulse oximeter working correctly? ✓ Presence of cardiac shunt ✓ Possibility of embolus	**D**islodged: Check ETT position • Mainstem • Not in trachea **O**bstructed: Suction ETT • Kinked • Mucus plug **P**neumothorax: Listen to breath sounds • Decompress with needle **E**quipment Check from patient to wall: • Oxygen flow • Valves • CO$_2$ canister • Inspect for disconnections and obstructions

HYPOXIA: LOSS OF ETCO$_2$
($\downarrow$ETCO$_2$ $\downarrow$SpO$_2$$\downarrow$BP)

Respiratory	Cardiac Output

Give 100% oxygen
Check:
✓ Airway patency
✓ Breathing circuit connections
   • Kinked endotracheal tube
✓ Breath sounds and chest excursion
   • Bilateral sounds and chest movement
   • Quality of breath sounds
   • Presence of **wheezing** or crackles
✓ Gas analyzer connections; power on ?
✓ Ventilation rate (excessive?)
	Embolus: air, blood, fat
	Actions: See "Air Embolism" card
	✓ Inform surgeon
	✓ Flood surgical field with saline
	✓ Lower surgical site below heart
	Low cardiac output or cardiac arrest
	Actions:
	✓ Follow PALS algorithm if cardiac arrest
	✓ Give 100% oxygen
	✓ Support ventilation
	✓ Support blood pressure with IV saline (10-20 mL/kg bolus)
	✓ Turn off anesthetic agents

LOCAL ANESTHETIC TOXICITY
(HYPOTENSION, RHYTHM DISTURBANCE, ALTERED CONSCIOUSNESS, SEIZURES)

- ✓ **Call for help.**
- ✓ **Stop local anesthetic.**
- ✓ Request **Intralipid** kit.
- ✓ Secure airway and ventilation.
- ✓ Give 100% oxygen.
- ✓ Confirm or establish adequate IV access.
- ✓ Confirm and monitor continuous ECG, BP, and SaO_2.
- ✓ Seizure treatment: **midazolam** 0.05-0.1 mg/kg IV or **propofol** 1-2 mg/kg IV. Treat resultant hypoventilation.
- ✓ Treat hypotension with small doses of **epinephrine** 1 µg/kg.
- ✓ Monitor and correct acidosis, hypercarbia, and hyperkalemia.
- ✓ **Avoid** vasopressin, calcium channel blockers, and beta blockers.
- ✓ If cardiac instability occurs:
  - Start **CPR.**
  - Start **Intralipid** therapy (see Intralipid Dosing)
    - Continue **chest compressions** (lipid must circulate).
- ✓ Consider alerting nearest cardiopulmonary bypass center and ICU if no ROSC.

INTRALIPID DOSING

- ✓ Bolus **Intralipid 20%** 1.5 mL/kg over 1 min.
- ✓ Start infusion 0.25 mL/kg/min.
- ✓ Repeat bolus every 3-5 min up to 3 mL/kg total dost until circulation is restored.
- ✓ Increase the rate to 0.5 mL/kg/min if BP remains low or declines.
- ✓ Continue infusion until hemodynamic stability is restored.
- ✓ Maximum total **Intralipid 20%** dose: 10 mL/kg over first 30 min.

LOSS OF EVOKED POTENTIALS
(MANAGEMENT OF SIGNAL CHANGES DURING SPINE SURGERY)

✓ Notify surgeon.
✓ Turn off inhalation agent/N_2O and switch to propofol/ketamine infusion.
✓ Turn off or reverse neuromuscular blockers.
✓ Increase perfusion pressure (MAP > 70 mm Hg) using ephedrine (0.2-0.3 mg/kg IV) and/or phenylephrine (1-10 µg/kg IV).
✓ Check Hb; transfuse RBC (10-15 mL/kg IV) if anemic.
✓ Ensure normocarbia: ↑ I/E ratio, ↓ PEEP.
✓ Ensure normothermia.
✓ Consider wake-up test.
✓ Consider high-dose steroid for spinal cord injury:
  • Methylprednisolone 30 mg/kg IV over 15 min, then 5.4 mg/kg/h IV infusion.

MALIGNANT HYPERTHERMIA
(⇑ TEMP, ⇑ HR, ⇑ CO_2, ACIDOSIS)

MH HOTLINE 1-800-644-9737

✓   **Call for help.**
✓   **Get Malignant Hyperthermia (MH) kit.**
✓   Stop procedure if possible.
✓   Stop volatile anesthetic. Transition to nontriggering anesthetic.
✓   Request chilled IV saline.
✓   **Hyperventilate** pt to reduce CO_2: 2-4 times patient's minute ventilation.
✓   **Dantrolene 2.5 mg/kg IV every 5 min** until symptoms resolve.
✓   Assign dedicated person to mix dantrolene (20 mg/vial) with 60 mL sterile water.
✓   **Bicarbonate 1-2 mEq/kg IV** for suspected metabolic acidosis; maintain pH > 7.2.
✓   **Cool patient** if temperature > 38.5°C.
  • NG lavage with cold water.
  • Apply ice externally.
  • Infuse cold saline intravenously.
    Stop cooling if temperature < 38°C.
✓   **Hyperkalemia treatment:** (See "Hyperkalemia" card.)
  • Ca gluconate 30 mg/kg IV or Ca chloride 10 mg/kg IV.
  • Sodium bicarbonate 1-2 mEq/kg IV.
  • Regular insulin 10 units IV with 1-2 amps D50 (0.1 unit insulin/kg and 1 mL/kg D50).
✓   **Dysrhythmia treatment:** Standard anti-arrhythmics; do **NOT** use calcium channel blocker.
✓   Send labs: ABG or VBG, electrolytes, serum CK, serum/urine myoglobin, coagulation.
✓   Place Foley catheter to monitor urine output.
✓   Call ICU to arrange disposition.

MYOCARDIAL ISCHEMIA
(ST CHANGES ON ECG)

RECOGNITION

✓ ST depression > 0.5 mm in any lead.
✓ ST elevation > 1 mm (2 mm in precordial lead).
✓ Flattened or inverted T waves.
✓ Arrhythmia: VF, VT, ventricular ectopy, heart block.

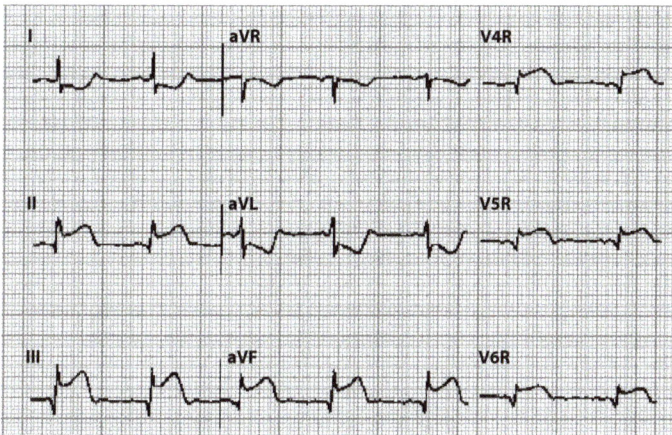

TREAT POTENTIAL CAUSES

✓ Severe hypoxemia
✓ Systemic arterial hypo- or hypertension
✓ Marked tachycardia
✓ Severe anemia
✓ Coronary air embolus
✓ Cardiogenic shock
✓ Local anesthetic toxicity

DIAGNOSTIC STUDIES

✓ 12-lead ECG:
  • II, III, aVF for inferior (RCA)
  • V5 for lateral ischemia (LCx)
  • V2, V3 anterior ischemia (LAD)
✓ Compare to previous ECGs
✓ Ped Cardiology consult; echocardiography

(continued on next page)

TREATMENT

✓ Improve O_2 supply.
  - 100% oxygen.
  - Correct anemia.
  - Correct hypotension.

✓ Decrease O_2 demand.
  - Reduce heart rate.
  - Correct hypertension.
  - Restore sinus rhythm.

✓ Drug therapy.
  - Nitroglycerin 0.5-5 µg/kg/min.
  - Consider heparin infusion.
    - 10 units/kg bolus, then 10 units/kg/h.

TACHYCARDIA
(TACHYCARDIA WITH PULSES, ASSOCIATED WITH HYPOTENSION)

DIAGNOSIS

✓ ST: narrow complex, P waves present before every QRS.
✓ SVT: narrow complex, no P waves or P waves not associated with QRS.
✓ VT: wide complex, polymorphic or monomorphic.

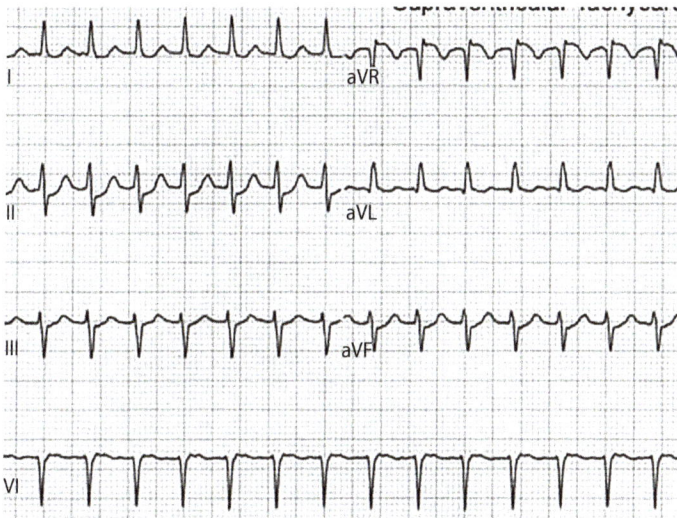

TREATMENT

If no pulse present, start CPR, go to "Cardiac Arrest, VF/VT" card
If pulse present:

Narrow Complex
✓ Vagal maneuvers: Ice to face; Valsalva; carotid massage.
✓ **Adenosine** 0.1-0.3 mg/kg IV push (max 1st dose 6 mg/max 2nd dose 12 mg).

Wide Complex
✓ Synchronized cardioversion at 0.5-1.0 J/kg (see table on next page).
✓ **Amiodarone** 5 mg/kg IV bolus over 20-60 min, *or*
✓ **Procainamide** 15 mg/kg IV bolus over 30-60 min, *or*
✓ **Lidocaine** 1 mg/kg IV bolus.

(*continued on next page*)

VT, Wide-Complex Irregular Rhythm	SVT, Tachyarrhythmias with Pulse
Biphasic 2 J/kg, then 4 J/kg for additional shocks	Synchronized cardioversion 0.5-1 J/kg, then 2 J/kg for additional shocks

Read Out H&Ts

Hypovolemia	Tension pneumothorax
Hypoxemia	Tamponade
Hydrogen ion	Thrombosis
(acidosis)	Toxin
Hyperkalemia	Trauma
Hypoglycemia	
Hypothermia	

TRANSFUSION: MASSIVE HEMORRHAGE
(REPLACEMENT OF > HALF OF TOTAL BLOOD VOLUME [TBV] PER HOUR OR TBV < 24 H)

✓ **Call for help.**
✓ Notify **blood bank** immediately of massive transfusion need.
  - **RBC : FFP : Platelets = 1:1:1.**
  - Use uncross-matched O negative blood until cross-matched blood available.
  - Give cryoprecipitate to maintain fibrinogen > 100.
✓ Obtain additional vascular access if needed.
✓ Send labs q30min.
  - Type and cross
  - CBC, platelets, PT/PTT/INR, fibrinogen
  - ABG, Na, K, Ca, lactate

✓ Warm the room.
✓ Blood product administration.
  - Use 140-micron filter for all products.
  - Use a blood warmer for RBC and FFP transfusion (not for platelets).
  - Rapid transfuser pumps may be used when increased flow is needed.
✓ Monitoring for hypothermia, hypocalcemia, electrolyte, blood gas, and acid-base disturbances.
✓ Consider rFactor Vlla for refractory hemorrhage if above measures are corrected.
✓ Terminate the massive transfusion protocol once bleeding is under control.

MAINTAIN

✓ HCT > 21% or HB > 7
✓ Platelet count > 50,000 (> 100k brain injury)
✓ INR < 1.5 (< 1.3 brain injury)
✓ Fibrinogen > 100

TRANSFUSION REACTIONS
(REACTIONS MAY OCCUR WITH ANY TYPE OF PRODUCT. IMPORTANT TO DETERMINE TYPE OF REACTION.)

FOR ALL REACTIONS

- ✓ **Call for help.**
- ✓ **Stop** transfusion.
- ✓ Disconnect donor product and IV tubing.
- ✓ Infuse normal saline through clean tubing.
- ✓ Examine blood product ID; determine correct pt.
- ✓ Send product to blood bank.
- ✓ Document per Institutional Policy

HEMOLYTIC—HGBEMIA, HGBURIA, DIC, ↓ BP, ↑ HR, BRONCHOSPASM

- ✓ Furosemide 0.1 mg/kg.
- ✓ Mannitol 0.5 g/kg (2 mL/kg of 25% mannitol).
- ✓ Dopamine (2-4 μg/kg/min).
- ✓ Maintain urine output at least 1-2 mL/kg/h.
- ✓ Prepare for cardiovascular instability.
- ✓ Send blood and urine sample to laboratory.

NONHEMOLYTIC—↓ BP, BRONCHOSPASM, PULMONARY EDEMA, FEVER, RASH

- ✓ Stop transfusion.
- ✓ Send blood to blood bank.
- ✓ Treat fever.
- ✓ Observe for signs of hemolysis.

ANAPHYLACTIC—ERYTHEMA, URTICARIA, ANGIOEDEMA, BRONCHOSPASM, TACHYCARDIA, SHOCK

- ✓ **Stop transfusion.**
- ✓ Support airway and circulation as necessary.
- ✓ Epinephrine 10 μg/kg IV.
- ✓ Diphenhydramine 1 mg/kg IV.
- ✓ Hydrocortisone 2-5 mg/kg.
- ✓ Maintain intravascular volume.

TRAUMA
(INITIAL MANAGEMENT OF TRAUMA)

PRIOR TO PT ARRIVAL TO OR

- ✓ Assemble team and assign roles.
- ✓ Estimate weight and prepare emergency drugs.
- ✓ Gather equipment:
  - Airway supplies
  - Invasive monitors
  - Fluid warmer
  - Rapid infusion device
  - Code cart with programmed defibrillator
- ✓ Type and cross blood products.

ON PT ARRIVAL TO OR

- ✓ Maintain c-spine precautions for transport.
- ✓ Secure/confirm airway (aspiration risk, unstable c-spine).
- ✓ Ensure adequate ventilation (maintain PIP <20 cm H_2o).
- ✓ Obtain/confirm large-bore IV access (central or interosseous if peripheral unsuccessful).
- ✓ Assess circulation.
- ✓ Persistent tachycardia, delayed cap refill, decreased pulse pressure = hypovolemia.
  - Bolus 20 mL/kg LR or NS (repeat × 2) and/or 10 mL/kg RBC or 20 mL/kg whole blood
- ✓ Place invasive monitors.
- ✓ Maintain normothermia.
- ✓ Rapidly treat associated conditions (acidosis, electrolyte disturbances).
- ✓ Continuously assess for secondary injury (ongoing blood loss).

HEAD TRAUMA
(INITIAL MANAGEMENT OF HEAD TRAUMA)

✓ Secure airway if GCS < 9, respiratory distress, hemodynamic instability, or elevated ICP.

✓ Maintain $PacO_2$ 30-35 mm Hg and PaO_2 > 60 mm Hg.

✓ Maintain cerebral perfusion pressure.
- (MAP – ICP) > 40 mm Hg and systolic BP > 5th percentile for age (see "Hypotension" card).
- Use CVP in place of ICP if no ICP monitor available.

✓ Treat elevated ICP with:
- Hyperventilation.
- Propofol or etomidate.
- Mannitol (1 g/kg).
- Hypertonic saline (3% via central venous catheter; 4 mL/kg).

✓ Maintain normoglycemia.
- Avoid glucose-containing solutions if hyperglycemic.

Note: Page numbers in *italics* refer to figures; page numbers followed by
t indicate tables.

www.ingramcontent.com/pod-product-compliance
Lightning Source LLC
Chambersburg PA
CBHW060800220326
41598CB00022B/2503